Theory & Practice of
THERAPEUTIC MASSAGE
Workbook
SIXTH EDITION

MARK F. BECK

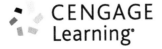

Australia • Brazil • Mexico • Singapore • United Kingdom • United States

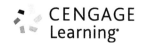
CENGAGE
Learning·

Theory & Practice of Therapeutic Massage Workbook, Sixth Edition
Mark F. Beck

Executive Director, Milady: Sandra Bruce

Product Director: Corina Santoro

Senior Content Developer: Jessica Mahoney

Product Assistant: Michelle Whitehead

Senior Director of Sales and Marketing:
  Gerard McAvey

Marketing Manager: Elizabeth Bushey

Senior Production Director: Wendy Troeger

Production Director: Andrew Crouth

Senior Content Project Manager:
  Nina Tucciarelli

Senior Art Director: Benj Gleeksman

Cover image(s): Image Source Photography /
  Veer.com

© 2017, 2011 Milady, a part of Cengage Learning

ALL RIGHTS RESERVED. No part of this work covered by the copyright herein may be reproduced or distributed in any form or by any means, except as permitted by U.S. copyright law, without the prior written permission of the copyright owner.

> For product information and technology assistance, contact us at
> **Cengage Learning Customer & Sales Support, 1-800-354-9706**
>
> For permission to use material from this text or product,
> submit all requests online at **www.cengage.com/permissions**.
> Further permissions questions can be e-mailed to
> **permissionrequest@cengage.com**

Library of Congress Control Number: 2016931122

ISBN-13: 978-1-285-18761-7

ISBN-10: 1-285-18761-X

Milady
20 Channel Center Street
Boston, MA 02210
USA

Cengage Learning is a leading provider of customized learning solutions with employees residing in nearly 40 different countries and sales in more than 125 countries around the world. Find your local representative at **www.cengage.com.**

Cengage Learning products are represented in Canada by Nelson Education, Ltd.

For your lifelong learning solutions, visit **www.milady.com**

Purchase any of our products at your local college store or at our preferred online store **www.cengagebrain.com**

Visit our corporate website at **cengage.com.**

Notice to the Reader
Publisher does not warrant or guarantee any of the products described herein or perform any independent analysis in connection with any of the product information contained herein. Publisher does not assume, and expressly disclaims, any obligation to obtain and include information other than that provided to it by the manufacturer. The reader is expressly warned to consider and adopt all safety precautions that might be indicated by the activities described herein and to avoid all potential hazards. By following the instructions contained herein, the reader willingly assumes all risks in connection with such instructions. The publisher makes no representations or warranties of any kind, including but not limited to, the warranties of fitness for particular purpose or merchantability, nor are any such representations implied with respect to the material set forth herein, and the publisher takes no responsibility with respect to such material. The publisher shall not be liable for any special, consequential, or exemplary damages resulting, in whole or part, from the readers' use of, or reliance upon, this material.

Printed at CLDPC, USA, 10-22

Contents

How to Use This Workbook

This *Theory & Practice of Therapeutic Massage Workbook* has been written to meet the needs, interests, and abilities of students, like you, receiving training in therapeutic massage.

This workbook should be used together with *Theory & Practice of Therapeutic Massage*, Sixth Edition. This workbook directly follows the information found in the student textbook.

Answer each item in this workbook with a pencil after consulting the textbook for the correct information. Items can be corrected and/or rated during class or individual discussions, or on an independent study basis.

A variety of question formats are included to emphasize essential facts found in the textbook and to measure your progress.

CHAPTER

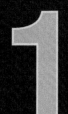

Historical Overview of Massage

FILL-IN-THE-BLANK: In the space(s) provided, write the word(s) that correctly complete(s) each statement.

1. The term *massage* was first used in American or European literature to denote using the hands to apply manipulations to the soft tissues during the _____ century.

2. Two terms the Chinese use for systems of massage are _____ and _____ .

3. There is documentation that the _____ have practiced massage since _____ .

4. The Japanese style of massage that uses finger pressure is _____ .

5. A sacred book of the Hindus written around 1800 BCE is the _____ .

6. The Hindu practice of bathing and massage that included kneading the extremities, tapotement, frictioning, anointing with perfumes, and cracking the joints of the fingers, toes, and the neck was known as _____ .

7. The _____ is a code of ethics for physicians and those about to receive medical degrees that bind them to honor their teachers, do their best to maintain the health of their patients, honor their patients' secrets, and prescribe no harmful treatment or drug.

8. The word that Hippocrates used to denote the art of rubbing upward, not downward, is _____ .

MATCHING: Match the name with the best description. Write the letter of that name in the space provided. Some names may be used more than once.

A. Asclepius
B. Avicenna
C. Celsus
D. Dr. James H. Cyriax
E. Elizabeth Dicke
F. Maria Ebner

G. Dr. Douglas O. Graham
H. Hippocrates
I. Albert J. Hoffa
J. Per Henrik Ling
K. Dr. Johann G. Mezger
L. Ambroise Paré

M. Mathias Roth
N. Charles Fayette Taylor
O. George Henry Taylor
P. Dr. Emil Vodder
Q. John Harvey Kellogg

_____ 1. Popularized use of the word *massage* in America

_____ 2. Credited with popularizing the terms *effleurage, petrissage, tapotement,* and *friction*

_____ 3. The Greek physician later worshipped as the "god of medicine"

_____ 4. The Greek physician who became known as the father of medicine

_____ 5. The name of the Roman physician who wrote *De Medicina*

_____ 6. The Persian philosopher/physician who wrote the *Canon of Medicine*

_____ 7. The French barber/surgeon who was one of the founders of modern surgery and who described in his publications the positive effects of medical rubbing in the healing process

_____ 8. Known as "the father of physical therapy"; developed a system of movements he called "medical gymnastics"

_____ 9. The English physician who published the first book in English on the Swedish movements

_____ 10. Established the first institute in England to teach Swedish movement gymnastics

_____ 11. Physician's brother who published the first American textbook on the Swedish movements

_____ 12. His use of the terms *effleurage, petrissage,* and *tapotement* are still in use today

_____ 13. A practitioner and historian who wrote about massage for more than 50 years and was a founding member of the American Physical Education Association

_____ 14. The distinguished German physician who published *Technik Der Massage*

_____ 15. The Austrian who developed a method of lymph massage

_____ 16. Developed *Bindegewebsmassage*

_____ 17. The New York physician who introduced the Swedish movements to the United States in 1858

_____ 18. An author, magazine editor, and the director of the Battle Creek Sanitarium

_____ 19. Popularized *Bindegewebsmassage* in England

_____ 20. The English orthopedic physician credited with popularizing deep transverse friction massage

MATCHING: Match the term with the best description. Write the letter of the appropriate term in the space provided.

A. acupressure   C. Rolfing   E. sports massage

B. reflexology   D. shiatsu   F. Swedish massage

_____ 1. Based on the Western concepts of anatomy and physiology, and uses effleurage, petrissage, vibration, friction, and tapotement

_____ 2. A method based on the traditional Oriental medical principles for assessing and treating the physical and energetic body order to regulate *chi* (the life force energy)

_____ 3. A finger-pressure method based on the Oriental concept that the body has a series of energy (*tsubo*) points

_____ 4. A method of massage especially designed to prepare an athlete for an upcoming event and to aid in the body's regenerative and restorative capacities following a rigorous workout or competition

_____ 5. Developed out of the technique of structural integration, it aligns the major body segments through manipulation of the fascia or the connective tissue

_____ 6. A method based on the idea that stimulation of particular points on the surface of the body has an effect on other areas or organs of the body

FILL-IN-THE-BLANK: In the space(s) provided, write the word(s) that correctly complete(s) each statement with regard to massage regulations.

1. The oldest professional massage organization in the United States is _____

   _____ .

2. The first time that massage was offered at the Summer Olympics was _____ .

3. Chair massage or seated massage was developed by _____ and introduced to the profession in the year _____ .

4. The agency in the United States recognized for certifying massage therapists is

_____ .

5. The agency named in No. 4 began testing and certifying massage therapists in the year

_____ .

6. Another phenomenon that was initiated in the 1990s that validates the effects and benefits of massage is _____ .

7. In the year _____ , the Federation of State Massage Therapy Boards formed to create a licensing examination called the _____ .

8. Numerous research projects that study the effects of touch on human well-being have been conducted at the _____ under the direction of Dr. Tiffany M. Fields.

9. The National Center for Complementary and Alternative Medicine was established in the year _____ by the _____ .

MULTIPLE CHOICE: Carefully read each statement. Choose the word or phrase that correctly completes the meaning and write the corresponding letter in the blank provided.

1. The system of ethical and professional application of structured, therapeutic touch to benefit soft-tissue health, movement, posture, and neurological patterns is called   _____
   a) shiatsu   c) physical therapy
   b) massage   d) chiropractic

2. Increased circulation, muscle relaxation, and pain relief are   _____
   a) problems of massage   c) medical conditions
   b) benefits of massage   d) massage movements

3. Massage has been part of Western medical traditions for at least   _____
   a) 10 years   c) 3,000 years
   b) 200 years   d) 10,000 years

4. Modern Chinese massage is called   _____
   a) *anmo*   c) *chi gong*
   b) shiatsu   d) *tuina*

5. The use of the term *massage* to denote the practice of manipulating the soft tissues first appeared in American literature around   _____
   a) 1890   c) 1774
   b) 1925   d) 1850

6. A finger-pressure technique used by the Japanese is called
   a) shiatsu
   b) *tui-na*
   c) *tsubo*
   d) acupuncture

7. The popularity of bathing and rubbing the body for health benefits lessened with the
   a) decline of the Roman Empire
   b) invention of hot tubs
   c) invention of electricity
   d) Inquisition

8. Much of Greco-Roman culture was preserved by the
   a) Spanish
   b) Romans
   c) Turks
   d) Persians

9. The father of physical therapy is
   a) Charles Fayette Taylor
   b) Hippocrates
   c) Asclepius
   d) Per Henrik Ling

10. The Swedish Movement Cure was brought to the United States by
    a) Douglas Graham
    b) Ambroise Paré
    c) the Taylor brothers
    d) Dr. Johann Mezger

11. The Greek physician who became known as the father of medicine was
    a) Homer
    b) Hippocrates
    c) Herodicus
    d) Asclepius

12. Much of modern massage terminology is based on terms from this language:
    a) Italian
    b) Chinese
    c) Greek
    d) French

13. Public interest in massage began to reemerge in the United States around
    a) 1950
    b) 1970
    c) 1960
    d) 1980

14. National certification in massage and bodywork has been available in the United States since
    a) 1961
    b) 1972
    c) 1985
    d) 1992

15. The idea that stimulation of particular body points affects other areas is called
    a) chiropractic
    b) reflexology
    c) Rolfing
    d) Trager

    _____

16. Neuromuscular techniques were developed in the 1940s by
    a) Dr. Leon Chaitow
    b) Paul St. John
    c) Boris Chaitow and Stanley Lief
    d) Janet Travell

    _____

17. A national organization that certifies massage therapists is the
    a) AMTA
    b) NCBTMB
    c) ABMP
    d) FSMTB

    _____

WORD REVIEW: Write down the meaning of each of the following words and titles. The list can be used later as a study guide for this chapter!

acupressure

_____

_____

_____

American Massage Therapy Association (AMTA)

_____

_____

_____

The American Organization for Bodywork Therapies of Asia (AOBTA)

_____

_____

_____

anatripsis

_____

_____

_____

Association of Bodywork Professionals (ABMP)

_____

_____

_____

Bindegewebsmassage

_____

_____

_____

bodywork

_____

_____

_____

chair massage

_____

_____

_____

chirurgy

_____

_____

_____

Connective Tissue Massage

_____

_____

_____

craniosacral therapy

_____

_____

_____

[1] Coalition of National Massage Therapy Organizations. (2013). _The core: Entry-level massage education blueprint_, pg. 57.

deep transverse friction massage

_____

_____

_____

Dr. Vodder's Manual Lymph Drainage

_____

_____

_____

effleurage

_____

_____

_____

Esalen massage

_____

_____

_____

Federation of State Massage Therapy Boards (FSMTB)

_____

_____

_____

Federation of Therapeutic Massage, Bodywork and Somatic Practice Organizations

_____

_____

_____

gymnasium

_____

_____

_____

Hippocratic Oath

_____

_____

_____

MBLEx

_____

_____

_____

manual lymph drainage

_____

_____

_____

massage

_____

_____

_____

_____

medical gymnastics

_____

_____

_____

National Center for Complementary and Alternative Medicine (NCCAM)

_____

_____

_____

National Certification Board for Therapeutic Massage and Bodywork (NCBTMB)

_____

_____

_____

neuromuscular therapy

_____

_____

_____

petrissage

_____

_____

_____

Polarity therapy

_____

_____

_____

reflexology

_____

_____

_____

Rolfing

_____

_____

_____

shiatsu

_____

_____

_____

sports massage

_____

_____

_____

Swedish Movement Cure

_____

_____

_____

tapotement

_____

_____

_____

Touch Research Institute

_____

_____

_____

Trager method

_____

_____

_____

Touch for Health

_____

_____

_____

tschanpua

_____

_____

_____

tsubo

_____

_____

_____

tuina

_____

_____

_____

CHAPTER

2

Requirements for the Practice of Therapeutic Massage

SHORT ANSWER: In the spaces provided, write short answers to the following questions.

1. What is meant by *scope of practice?*

   _____

   _____

2. In states that have massage licensing, how is the scope of practice defined?

   _____

   _____

3. In the United States, which jurisdiction might oversee regulations for massage?

   _____

   _____

4. What is the major reason for licensing massage therapists?

   _____

   _____

5. What is the role of state regulatory boards?

   _____

   _____

6. What are the requirements for licensure in most states?

   _____

   _____

TRUE OR FALSE: If the following statements are true, write *true* in the space provided. If they are false, write *false*.

_____ 1. If a massage therapist is nationally certified, she can practice anywhere in the United States.

_____ 2. If a massage therapist has a license in one state, they can legally practice in a neighboring state.

_____ 3. In a state that has massage licensing, if a licensed nurse or chiropractor wants to practice massage, she must obtain a massage license.

_____ 4. The scope of practice for massage is clearly defined by national standards.

SHORT ANSWER: Of the following statements, put a check mark in front of the ones that may be grounds for revoking, canceling, or suspending a massage license.

_____ 1. Having been convicted of a felony

_____ 2. Being guilty of fraudulent or deceptive advertising

_____ 3. Being engaged currently or previously in any act of prostitution

_____ 4. Practicing under a false or assumed name

_____ 5. Being accused of making sexual advances or attempting sexual acts during the course of a massage

_____ 6. Prescribing drugs or medicines (unless you are a licensed physician)

_____ 7. Charging extremely high fees for the services provided

_____ 8. Being addicted to narcotics, alcohol, or like substances that interfere with the performance of duties

_____ 9. Being guilty of fraud or deceit in obtaining a license

_____ 10. Selling nutritional products or other non-massage-related items

_____ 11. Being willfully negligent in the practice of massage so as to endanger the health of a client

FILL-IN-THE-BLANK: In the space(s) provided, write the word(s) that correctly complete(s) each statement.

1. A _____ is issued by a state or municipal regulating agency as a requirement for conducting a business or practicing a trade or profession.

2. A document that is awarded in recognition of an accomplishment or for achieving or maintaining some kind of standard is a _____ .

3. Ongoing training that is required to renew a license or certification is termed _____ .

MULTIPLE CHOICE: Carefully read each statement. Choose the word or phrase that correctly completes the meaning and write the corresponding letter in the blank provided.

1. *Scope of practice* defines _____
   a) legally acceptable professional activities
   b) medical ethics
   c) specific techniques
   d) geographical boundaries

2. If a client's condition is outside the massage technician's scope of practice, the technician should _____
   a) schedule extra sessions
   b) refer the client to the proper professional
   c) take more training
   d) refer to textbooks

3. The main reason for massage licensing is _____
   a) to make sure that people who only graduate from special schools practice
   b) to ensure that only certain kinds of massage are practiced
   c) to protect the safety of the public
   d) to close down massage studios

4. Testing and licensing of massage professionals is generally overseen by _____
   a) a regulatory board
   b) the legislature
   c) a professional massage association
   d) a local law enforcement agency

5. Being licensed in one city or state _____ validation in another location.
   a) does not guarantee
   b) requires
   c) guarantees
   d) assumes

6. The minimum education requirement for the National Certification for Therapeutic Massage and Bodywork Board Certification is
   a) 300 hours
   b) 250 hours
   c) 1,000 hours
   d) 750 hours

7. A document awarded in recognition of achieving or maintaining a set standard is a
   a) recommendation
   b) license
   c) certificate
   d) diploma

8. Completing a course of study or passing an examination results in
   a) certification
   b) licensing
   c) a diploma
   d) job security

9. Certificates can be awarded by all the following except
   a) schools
   b) professional organizations
   c) institutions
   d) governmental agency

10. A document issued by a regulatory agency that is required to practice a trade or profession is a
    a) certification
    b) permit
    c) ordinance
    d) license

11. A document awarded for achieving or maintaining some standard or accomplishment is a
    a) commendation
    b) certificate
    c) license
    d) promotion

12. *Scope of practice* is defined in
    a) textbooks
    b) licensing regulations
    c) professional organizations
    d) medical dictionary

FILL-IN-THE-BLANK: In the space(s) provided, write the word(s) that correctly complete(s) each statement.

1. A systemized and organized attempt to test if a hypothesis has validity is

   _____ .

2. A practice that is based on client's wishes, clinical experience, and current scientific evidence is said to be _____ .

3. Phrases or words to help in the search for relative articles are known as

   _____ .

4. A condensed version of a research paper that includes background, objectives for the report, case presentation, and discussion of the results is called an _____ .

5. Research involving a number of subjects randomly divided into treatment groups, one being a control group and others receiving treatments, so that comparisons can be made regarding the effectiveness of treatment is known as _____ .

6. When two or more of the studies referred to in question six are confined and statistically analyzed, it is called a _____ .

PRIORITIZE: Prioritize the research methodology from highest to the lowest reliability, by placing the letters A to E in front of the term (A being the highest reliability and E being the lowest).

1. _____ Preliminary research

2. _____ Clinical experience

3. _____ Randomized controlled trial

4. _____ Meta-analysis

5. _____ Case report

MATCHING: Match the term with the best description of the sections of a case report. Write the letter of the appropriate term in the space provided.

A. abstract
B. results

C. introduction
D. discussion

E. presentation
F. references

_____ 1. Provides bibliographic information.

_____ 2. Provides the methodological details.

_____ 3. A condensed version of a research paper.

_____ 4. Provides background information so the reader can understand the topic.

_____ 5. Provides a summary and meaning to the results.

_____ 6. Presents the findings of the project without interpretation.

WORD REVIEW: Write down the meaning of each of the following words and titles. The list can be used later as a study guide for this chapter!

Certification

_____

_____

_____

continuing education

_____

_____

_____

license

_____

_____

_____

evidence-informed practice

_____

_____

_____

Board Certified Examination for Therapeutic Massage and Bodywork (BCETMB)

_____

_____

_____

_____

_____

scope of practice

_____

_____

_____

CHAPTER 3

Professional Ethics for Massage Practitioners

FILL-IN-THE-BLANK: In the space(s) provided, write the word(s) from the following list that correctly complete(s) each statement.

confidential

courtesy

ethics

fairness

honest

professional

a satisfied customer

sexual

tactful

1. The standards and philosophy of human conduct or code of morals of an individual, group, or profession is known as _____.

2. One of the best forms of advertising in a personal service business is _____.

3. A person engaged in a vocation or occupation requiring advanced training to gain knowledge and skills is considered a _____.

4. All clients should be treated with _____ and _____.

5. All communications with clients should be _____ and _____.

6. Be respectful of the therapeutic relationship and maintain appropriate _____ boundaries.

7. To handle a client who is overly critical, finds fault, and is hard to please, the therapist must be _____.

MATCHING: Match the term with the best description. Write the letter of the appropriate term in the space provided.

A. personal boundary   D. dual relationship   G. countertransference

B. professional boundary   E. power differential   H. supervision

C. therapeutic relationship   F. transference

_____ 1. A client-centered relationship in which all activities benefit and enhance the client's well-being

_____ 2. A relationship in which one person is more vulnerable

_____ 3. Defined by our experiences, beliefs, and upbringing

_____ 4. Practitioner personalizes the relationship with the client

_____ 5. Practice that protects the client and the therapist

_____ 6. A shame-free environment in which to sort out emotional or boundary issues

_____ 7. Client projects attributes of someone from a former relationship onto the practitioner

_____ 8. A social or romantic relationship outside or beyond the therapeutic relationship

_____ 9. Practitioner-client relationship free of physical, emotional, or sexual impropriety

_____ 10. Parent-child, therapist-client, teacher-student relationships exhibit this characteristic

_____ 11. Provide a framework to function safely in the world

_____ 12. Client seeks more out of the relationship than is therapeutically appropriate

_____ 13. Creates a safe environment and stable framework from which to practice

_____ 14. Unconscious phenomena that occur in therapeutic relationships in which there is a power differential

_____ 15. A secondary relationship that extends beyond the massage practitioner-client relationship

_____ 16. Conferring with a mentor, a colleague, or a peer group regarding ethical issues

SHORT ANSWER: In the spaces provided, write short answers to the following questions.

1. List nine attributes that are helpful for developing good human relations between therapist and client.

   a. _____

   b. _____

   c. _____

   d. _____

   e. _____

   f. _____

   g. _____

   h. _____

   i. _____

2. The most effective tool to prevent or clarify boundary issues is

   _____ .

3. List eight major areas to consider when establishing professional boundaries.

   a. _____

   b. _____

   c. _____

   d. _____

   e. _____

   f. _____

   g. _____

   h. _____

MULTIPLE CHOICE: Carefully read each statement. Choose the word or phrase that correctly completes the meaning and write the corresponding letter in the blank provided.

1. The code of morals of a profession, group, or individual person is called _____
   a) values
   b) attitudes
   c) morals
   d) ethics

2. A person in an occupation that requires advanced training to gain skills and knowledge is considered a _____
   a) journeyman
   b) professional
   c) skilled laborer
   d) veteran

3. A massage therapist's best method of advertising is _____
   a) satisfied clients
   b) newspaper
   c) radio
   d) Internet

4. Intimate or sexual relationships between client and practitioner are _____
   a) avoided
   b) done only with full consent
   c) not done in the massage facility
   d) done only for therapeutic reasons

5. A situation where the therapist has a social relationship with a client is _____
   a) countertransference
   b) known as transference
   c) called supervision
   d) a dual relationship

6. Professional standards are determined by educational requirements, codes of ethics, and _____
   a) standards of practice
   b) scope of practice
   c) state and local regulations
   d) all of the above

7. Guidelines that help to define us emotionally and spiritually, are determined by our experiences and beliefs, and act as a safety net and personal protection are _____
   a) personal boundaries
   b) codes of ethics
   c) morals
   d) professional boundaries

8. _____ are preliminarily outlined in policy and procedure statements and protect the safety of the client and the therapist. _____
   a) Codes of ethics
   b) Professional boundaries
   c) Standards of practice
   d) Personal boundaries

9. A(n) _____ relationship is a practitioner-client relationship that is client centered, in which all activities are to benefit and enhance the client's well-being and maintain or promote his or her welfare. _____
   a) intimate
   c) therapeutic
   b) unhealthy
   d) medical

10. In a practitioner-client relationship, the foundation that provides an environment of safety, trust, and respect for the client to relax, open, release, and heal is _____
   a) confidentiality
   c) clear policies and procedures
   b) a thorough assessment
   d) being well educated

11. A relationship in which more authority is held by the person on one side of the relationship, whereas the other person is in a more vulnerable or submissive role is _____
   a) an abusive relationship
   c) a power differential
   b) a therapeutic relationship
   d) countertransference

12. When a client unconsciously projects attributes of someone from a former relationship onto a therapist or seeks more out of the relationship than is therapeutically appropriate, it is called _____
   a) countertransference
   c) fantasizing
   b) projecting
   d) transference

13. When a practitioner begins to personalize or take a therapeutic relationship with the client personally it is called _____
   a) transference
   c) countertransference
   b) a power differential
   d) unethical

14. Any situation that combines the therapeutic relationship with a secondary relationship that extends beyond the massage practitioner-client relationship is _____
   a) unethical
   c) a dual relationship
   b) therapeutic
   d) illegal

15. In a therapeutic relationship, whose responsibility is it to maintain appropriate boundaries? _____
   a) the therapist or practitioner
   c) both the client and the therapist
   b) the client
   d) all of the above

16. When a therapist becomes involved in instances of transference, countertransference, or dual relationships, she should _____
   a) discontinue the relationship
   c) feel ashamed
   b) quit her practice
   d) seek supervision

WORD REVIEW: Write down the meaning of each of the following words and titles. The list can be used later as a study guide for this chapter!

boundaries

_____

_____

_____

Code of Ethics

_____

_____

_____

confidentiality

_____

_____

_____

countertransference

_____

_____

_____

dual relationship

_____

_____

_____

duty to warn and protect

_____

_____

_____

ethics

_____

_____

_____

personal boundaries

_____

_____

_____

power differential

_____

_____

_____

professional

_____

_____

_____

professionalism

_____

_____

_____

professional boundaries

_____

_____

_____

supervision

_____

_____

_____

therapeutic relationship

_____

_____

_____

transference

_____

_____

_____

CHAPTER

4

Overview of Human Anatomy and Physiology and Medical Terminology

FILL-IN-THE-BLANK: In the space(s) provided, write the word(s) that correctly complete(s) each statement.

1. The study of the gross structure of the body or the study of an organism and the interrelations of its parts is _____ .

2. The science and study of the vital processes, mechanisms, and functions of an organ or system of organs is _____ .

3. The study of the structural and functional changes caused by disease is _____ .

4. The scientific study of muscular activity and the mechanics of body movement is _____ .

5. The delicate physiologic balance that the body strives to maintain in its internal environment is _____.

6. The abnormal and unhealthy state of all or part of the body where it is incapable of carrying on its normal function is _____ .

7. A _____ of a disease is perceived by the victim, whereas a _____ of a disease is observable by another person.

KEY CHOICES: Massage can have a direct, an indirect, or a reflex effect on various functions of the body. Put the appropriate key letter for each of the following phrases in the spaces provided.

D = Direct effect

I = Indirect effect

R = Reflex effect

_____ 1. Increased circulation to the muscle and internal organs

_____ 2. Stretching of muscle tissue

_____ 3. Slower, deeper breathing

_____ 4. Loosening of adhesions and scar tissue

_____ 5. Reduced heart rate

_____ 6. Reduced blood pressure

_____ 7. Increased local circulation of venous blood

_____ 8. General relaxation of tense muscles

KEY CHOICES: Most diseases have signs and/or symptoms. Put the appropriate key letter for each of the following phrases in the spaces provided.

X = Symptom

O = Sign

_____ 1. nausea

_____ 2. abnormal skin color

_____ 3. pain

_____ 4. chills

_____ 5. elevated pulse

_____ 6. severe itching

_____ 7. abdominal cramps

_____ 8. fever

_____ 9. dizziness

_____ 10. skin ulcers

FILL-IN-THE-BLANK: In the space(s) provided, write the word(s) that correctly complete(s) each statement.

1. Two hormones that are secreted by the adrenal glands are _____ and
_____.

2. The protective body sensation that warns of tissue damage or destruction
is _____.

3. The two reactions to pain are _____ and _____.

4. Inhibited blood flow to an area of the body is known as _____.

5. A syndrome that often starts as a simple muscle spasm that is complicated by muscle splinting
and constricted circulation is the _____.

6. Much of the discomfort in the condition of the previous question is from
_____.

7. Psychologically, skillfully applied therapeutic massage helps to reduce pain by relieving
_____ and _____.

8. In a pain–spasm–pain cycle, pain is intensified because of _____.

9. Therapeutic massage on contracted ischemic tissue relieves _____ and
restores _____.

10. Pain is an indication of _____ or _____.

11. Generally, the more severe the pain, the more severe the _____.

12. Bacteria, viruses, fungi, and parasites are _____.

13. If pathogenic organisms enter the body in large enough numbers to multiply and become
capable of destroying healthy tissue, they cause _____.

14. If these organisms are confined to a small area, the condition is considered a
_____, but if they spread throughout the body, the condition is termed a
_____.

15. When tissue is damaged from invading organisms or physical injury, substances are released
that cause _____.

16. Inflammation is a protective tissue response characterized by _____,
_____, _____, and _____.

17. An elevated body temperature that accompanies infectious diseases is a _____.

18. The fibrous connective tissue formed as a wound heals is _____.

19. Connective tissue fibers are produced in healing tissue by _____.

SHORT ANSWER: In the spaces provided, write short answers to the following questions.

1. List six possible direct causes of disease.

    a. _____

    b. _____

    c. _____

    d. _____

    e. _____

    f. _____

2. Stress is most notably associated with the adrenal glands and their secretion of the "fight-or-flight" hormones. Briefly describe what happens to the following body functions during the "fight-or-flight" reaction.

    1. Muscle tone _____

    2. Blood pressure _____

    3. Digestion _____

    4. Circulation to skeletal muscles _____

    5. Circulation to digestive organs _____

    6. Red blood cells _____

FILL-IN-THE-BLANK: In the space(s) provided, write the word(s) that correctly complete(s) each statement.

1. Physiologically, skillfully applied therapeutic massage helps to reduce pain by providing

    _____

    _____ .

2. If massage increases the overall intensity of the pain, the therapist should _____

    _____ .

3. A wellness-oriented person attempts to maintain a balance between _____ ,
    _____ , and _____ .

4. In medical terminology, compound words are constructed of _____ ,
    _____ , and _____ .

MATCHING: In the following six exercises match the term in the first column with the meaning in the second column. Write the letter of the appropriate term in the space provided.

WORD ROOTS I

_____	1. arth(ro)	A.	lung
_____	2. chondr/o	B.	tissue
_____	3. cyt	C.	joint
_____	4. hem	D.	nerve
_____	5. hist	E.	cell
_____	6. my(o)	F.	heat
_____	7. neur(o)	G.	blood
_____	8. oss, ost(e)	H.	vessel
_____	9. phleb	I.	bone
_____	10. pulmo	J.	cartilage
_____	11. therm	K.	vein
_____	12. vas	L.	muscle

WORD ROOTS II

_____	1. brachi	A.	head
_____	2. cardi	B.	kidney
_____	3. cephal	C.	foot
_____	4. derm	D.	stomach
_____	5. gastr(o)	E.	arm
_____	6. gyn	F.	woman
_____	7. hepat	G.	skin
_____	8. labi	H.	lung
_____	9. nephr(o)	I.	liver
_____	10. ocul	J.	heart
_____	11. pneum	K.	eye
_____	12. pod	L.	lip

PREFIXES I

_____ 1. ab-

_____ 2. ad-

_____ 3. anti-

_____ 4. ante-

_____ 5. bio-

_____ 6. contra-

_____ 7. ex-

_____ 8. infra-

_____ 9. extra-

_____ 10. intra-

_____ 11. sub-

_____ 12. super-

A. beyond, outside of, in addition

B. against

C. against, counter to

D. away from

E. inside

F. above, in addition

G. before

H. out of

I. to, toward

J. beneath

K. under, below

L. life

PREFIXES II

_____ 1. ect-

_____ 2. end-(o)

_____ 3. epi-

_____ 4. hyper-

_____ 5. hypo-

_____ 6. mega-

_____ 7. micr-(o)

_____ 8. mon-(o)

_____ 9. narc-

_____ 10. path-

_____ 11. peri-

_____ 12. pseud(o)

A. under, below

B. one, single

C. inside, within

D. around

E. stupor, numbness

F. upon, over, in addition

G. large, extreme

H. outside, without

I. pertaining to disease

J. small

K. false

L. above, extreme

PREFIXES III

_____ 1. hemi-

_____ 2. hetero-

_____ 3. hom-

_____ 4. medi-

_____ 5. multi-

_____ 6. para-

_____ 7. poly-

_____ 8. quad-

_____ 9. retro-

_____ 10. syn-

_____ 11. tri-

_____ 12. uni-

A. many, much

B. middle, midline

C. the other

D. together, along with

E. four

F. single, one

G. common, same

H. many, multiple

I. half

J. three

K. next to, resembling, beside

L. backward

SUFFIXES

_____ 1. -ase

_____ 2. -algia

_____ 3. -ectomy

_____ 4. -graph

_____ 5. -ia

_____ 6. -itis

_____ 7. -ology

_____ 8. -oma

_____ 9. -ostomy

_____ 10. -otomy

_____ 11. -pathic

_____ 12. -phobia

A. diseased

B. study of, science of

C. forming an opening

D. surgical removal of body part

E. denoting an enzyme

F. tumor

G. write, draw, record

H. morbid fear of

I. excision, cutting into

J. painful condition

K. inflammation

L. a noun ending of a condition

MULTIPLE CHOICE: Carefully read each statement. Choose the word or phrase that correctly completes the meaning and write the corresponding letter in the blank provided.

1. The scientific study of body movement is
   a) anatomy
   b) kinesiology
   c) pathology
   d) physiology

2. Normal functions of body systems are studied in
   a) physiology
   b) histology
   c) anatomy
   d) pathology

3. The study of the gross structure of the body or an organism and its parts is known as
   a) physiology
   b) histology
   c) anatomy
   d) pathology

4. Describing how the organs or body parts function and relate to one another is
   a) physiology
   b) histology
   c) anatomy
   d) pathology

5. The study of structural and functional changes caused by disease is
   a) physiology
   b) histology
   c) anatomy
   d) pathology

6. Lower blood pressure and general relaxation are _____ effects of massage.
   a) recurring
   b) indirect
   c) direct
   d) reflex

7. The body's internal balance is called
   a) blood chemistry
   b) breathing
   c) homeostasis
   d) physiology

8. Perceived conditions such as dizziness, nausea, or pain are called
   a) symptoms
   b) diseases
   c) homeostasis
   d) signs

9. Observable indications such as fever, abnormal pulse rate, or abnormal skin color are
   a) symptoms of disease
   b) illnesses
   c) signs of disease
   d) psychosomatic

10. The adrenal hormone that acts as an anti-inflammatory and antiallergenic in stressful situations is
    a) DMSO
    b) cortisol
    c) estrogen
    d) adrenaline

    _____

11. Prolonged adrenal excretions make the body
    a) exhausted
    b) energetic
    c) strong
    d) ecstatic

    _____

12. The pain–spasm–pain cycle is associated with
    a) headaches
    b) heart attacks
    c) muscle spasms
    d) mental health

    _____

13. The condition in which contracted muscles inhibit blood flow to an area is called
    a) constriction
    b) ischemia
    c) hypertension
    d) bruising

    _____

14. The existence of disease-producing organisms throughout the body is termed a/an
    a) microorganism
    b) inflammation
    c) systemic infection
    d) local infection

    _____

15. A protective tissue response characterized by swelling, redness, heat, and pain is
    a) ischemia
    b) spasm
    c) sunburn
    d) inflammation

    _____

16. In medical terminology, the root word usually indicates the
    a) number
    b) body part
    c) condition
    d) treatment

    _____

17. The medical-term prefix *a* means
    a) one
    b) many
    c) without
    d) after

    _____

18. The medical-term prefix *ambi* means
    a) in twos
    b) both
    c) walking
    d) movement

    _____

19. The medical-term prefix *infra* means
    a) beneath   c) inside
    b) above   d) outside   _____

20. The medical-term suffix *algia* means
    a) three   c) inflammation
    b) binding   d) painful condition _____

21. The medical-term suffix *itis* means
    a) inflammation   c) resembling
    b) old   d) tumor   _____

22. The medical-term suffix *pathic* means
    a) germs   c) toxic
    b) tumor   d) diseased   _____

23. The medical term root *arth(ro)* means
    a) joint   c) blood
    b) bone   d) lung   _____

24. The medical term root *derm* means
    a) teeth   c) skin
    b) bone   d) lung   _____

WORD REVIEW: Write down the meaning of each of the following words and titles. The list can be used later as a study guide for this chapter!

adrenaline

_____

_____

_____

anatomy

_____

_____

_____

atherosclerosis

_____

_____

_____

bacteria

_____

_____

_____

cortisol

_____

_____

_____

disease

_____

_____

_____

fever

_____

_____

_____

fungus

_____

_____

_____

homeostasis

_____

_____

_____

infection

_____

_____

_____

inflammation

_____

_____

_____

ischemia

_____

_____

_____

ischemic pain

_____

_____

_____

kinesiology

_____

_____

_____

local infection

_____

_____

_____

medical terminology

_____

_____

_____

microorganisms

_____

_____

_____

pain

_____

_____

_____

pain–spasm–pain cycle

_____

_____

_____

parasite

_____

_____

_____

pathology

_____

_____

_____

physiology

_____

_____

_____

scar tissue

_____

_____

_____

sign of disease

_____

_____

_____

stress

_____

_____

_____

symptom

_____

_____

_____

systemic infection

_____

_____

_____

virus

_____

_____

_____

wellness

_____

_____

_____

CHAPTER

5 Human Anatomy and Physiology

INTRODUCTION

FILL-IN-THE-BLANK: In the space(s) provided, write the word(s) that correctly complete(s) each statement.

1. The submicroscopic particles that make up all substances are called _____.

2. These are arranged in specific patterns and structures called _____.

3. In the human organism, the basic unit of structure and function is the _____.

4. These are organized into layers or groups called _____.

5. Groups of these form complex structures that perform certain functions. These structures are called _____ and are arranged in _____.

6. All living matter is composed of a colorless, jelly-like substance called _____.

7. The cytoplasm contains a network of various membranes called _____, which perform specific functions necessary for cell survival.

8. The type of cell division that takes place in the sex glands to create the sperm and egg is _____.

9. During the early developmental stages of an organism, the repeated division of the ovum results in many specialized cells that differ from one another in composition and function. This process is called _____.

10. In the human organism, as a cell matures and is nourished, it grows in size and eventually divides into two smaller cells. This form of cell division is called _____.

SHORT ANSWER: In the spaces provided, write short answers to the following questions.

1. In order to grow and function, a cell requires:

   a. _____   c. _____

   b. _____   d. _____

2. Name the four principal parts of a cell.

   a. _____   c. _____

   b. _____   d. _____

MATCHING: Match each term with its associated function. Write the letter of the appropriate term in the space provided.

A. cell membrane	F. Golgi apparatus	K. nucleolus
B. centrosome	G. lysosome	L. nucleus
C. chromatin	H. microtubules	M. ribosome
D. endoplasmic reticulum	I. mitochondria	N. vacuole
E. fibrils	J. nuclear membrane	

_____ 1. converts and releases energy for cell operation

_____ 2. contains cellular material and transports materials between the inside and outside of the cell

_____ 3. produce lipids or proteins for cell utilization and transport

_____ 4. stores the body's genetic code

_____ 5. synthesizes carbohydrates and holds protein for secretion

_____ 6. involved in the rapid introduction or ejection of substances

_____ 7. divides and moves to opposite poles of the cell during mitosis

_____ 8. controls passage of substances between the nucleus and cytoplasm

_____ 9. composed of RNA and protein molecules that synthesize proteins

_____ 10. fibers of protein and DNA that contain the genes

IDENTIFICATION: Identify the structures indicated in Figure 5-1 by writing the letter of the structure next to the appropriate name in the space provided.

_____ 1. cell membrane

_____ 2. chromatin

_____ 3. smooth endoplasmic reticulum

_____ 4. Golgi apparatus

_____ 5. lysosome

_____ 6. pinocytic vesicle

_____ 7. mitochondria

_____ 8. nucleolus

_____ 9. nucleus

_____ 10. ribosomes

_____ 11. vacuole

_____ 12. rough endoplasmic reticulum

_____ 13. cytoplasm

_____ 14. centrioles

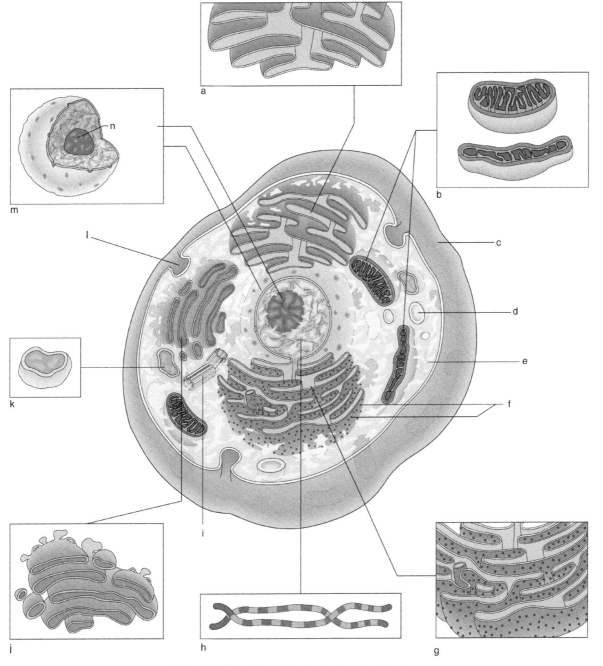

Fig. 5-1 Structure of a typical animal cell.

SHORT ANSWER: The five phases of cell division are listed next. Number the phases from 1 to 5 to indicate the correct order in which they occur.

_____ metaphase   _____ interphase   _____ anaphase

_____ telophase   _____ prophase

MATCHING: Match the term with the best description. Write the letter of the best description in the space provided

_____ 1. metaphase

_____ 2. telophase

_____ 3. interphase

_____ 4. prophase

_____ 5. anaphase

A. Chromosomes become larger and can be seen as two coiled strands called *chromatids*.

B. This is the normal state of the cell during growth.

C. Cytoplasm divides into two cells.

D. Chromosomes arrange along the equatorial plane.

E. The chromatids are separated and are again called *chromosomes*.

FILL-IN-THE-BLANK: In the space(s) provided, write the word(s) that correctly complete(s) each statement.

1. The chemical reactions within a cell that transform food into nutrients used for cell growth and operation are broadly termed _____.

2. Two phases of metabolism are _____ and _____.

3. The process of building up larger molecules from smaller ones is _____.

4. The process of breaking down larger substances or molecules into smaller ones is

_____.

5. Protein substances that act as organic catalysts to initiate, accelerate, or control specific chemical reactions in the metabolic process are called _____.

6. Collections of similar cells that carry out specific functions of the body are called

_____.

SHORT ANSWER: In the spaces provided, list the four main categories of tissues.

1. _____

2. _____

3. _____

4. _____

IDENTIFICATION: In the space provided, write the name of the tissue type that best fits the description.

_____ 1. represented by blood and lymph

_____ 2. functions in the process of absorption, excretion, secretion, and protection

_____ 3. binds structures together and serves as a framework

_____ 4. acts as a channel for the transmission of messages

_____ 5. forms the skin, the covering of the organs, and the inner lining of all the hollow organs

_____ 6. carries nutrients to the cells and carries away waste products

_____ 7. deep fascia, superficial fascia

_____ 8. initiates, controls, and coordinates the body's adaptation to its surroundings

_____ 9. contracts and causes movement

_____ 10. always has a free surface that is exposed to outside influences

_____ 11. responsible for the movement of food through the digestive tract, the constriction of blood vessels, and the emptying of the bladder

_____ 12. bones, cartilage, and ligaments

_____ 13. cells classified by shape as squamous, cuboidal, and columnar

_____ 14. provides support and protection

_____ 15. covers all the surfaces of the body

_____ 16. responsible for pumping blood through the heart into the blood vessels

_____ 17. composed of neurons

_____ 18. makes up the major tissue of the glands

_____ 19. responsible for facial expression, speaking, and other voluntary movements

FILL-IN-THE-BLANK: In the space(s) provided, write the word(s) that correctly complete(s) each statement.

1. Two categories of membranes are _____ membranes and _____membranes.

2. _____ produce a thick, sticky substance that acts as a protectant and lubricant.

3. _____ produce a watery, lubricating substance that lines the body cavities and sometimes forms the outermost surface of the organs contained in those cavities.

4. Three major serous membranes are the _____ that encases the lungs, the _____ around the heart, and the _____ that lines the abdominal cavity.

SHORT ANSWER: In the spaces provided, write short answers to the following questions.

1. List three fascial layers associated with the muscles.

   a. _____

   b. _____

   c. _____

2. Name three types of skeletal membrane and state where each is found.

   a. _____

   b. _____

   c. _____

MATCHING: Match the term with the best description. Write the letter of the best description in the space provided.

_____ 1. elastic cartilage

_____ 2. areolar tissue

_____ 3. Bone or osseous tissue

_____ 4. adipose tissue

_____ 5. ligaments

_____ 6. fibrocartilage

_____ 7. dense connective tissue

A. impregnated with mineral salts, chiefly calcium phosphate and calcium carbonate

B. found between the vertebrae and in the pubic symphysis

C. found in the external ear and the larynx

D. found on the ends of bones and in movable joints

E. fibrous bands that connect bones to bones

F. composed of collagen and elastic fibers that are closely arranged

_____ 8. tendons

G. cords or bands that serve to attach muscle to bone

_____ 9. hyaline cartilage

H. binds the skin to the underlying tissues and fills the spaces between the muscles

I. has an abundance of fat-containing cells

FILL-IN-THE-BLANK: In the space(s) provided, write the word(s) that correctly complete(s) each statement.

1. The three types of muscle tissue are _____, _____, and _____.

2. _____ are usually attached to bone or other muscle by way of tendons, and they can be controlled by conscious effort.

3. Because these muscles have alternating light and dark cross markings, they are called _____.

4. Muscle tissue found in the hollow organs of the stomach, small intestine, colon, bladder, and the blood vessels does not have the cross markings and is called _____ or _____ muscle.

5. _____ is found only in the heart.

MULTIPLE CHOICE: Carefully read each statement. Choose the word or phrase that correctly completes the meaning and write the corresponding letter in the blank provided.

1. All substances are made from subatomic particles that form _____.   _____

   a) molecules   c) atoms
   b) tissues   d) cells

2. The basic structure in human organisms is the _____.   _____
   a) organ   c) cell
   b) tissue   d) molecule

3. Cell division, which produces new identical daughter cells, is called _____.   _____

   a) mutation   c) amitosis
   b) mitosis   d) gestation

4. The complex chemical and physical process that nourishes organisms is called _____.
   a) mitosis
   b) metabolism
   c) homeostasis
   d) nutrition

5. Microscopic structures in the cytoplasm of the cell that produce energy needed for cellular work are called _____.
   a) lysosomes
   b) mitochondria
   c) Golgi bodies
   d) endoplasmic reticulum

6. Anabolism and catabolism are closely regulated to maintain

   _____.

   a) prophase
   b) enzymes
   c) amitosis
   d) homeostasis

7. Which of the following is not one of the four main human tissue types? _____.
   a) epithelial
   b) connective
   c) nervous
   d) skeletal

8. A special molecule that stores energy for use in muscular activity is

   _____.

   a) adenosine triphosphate
   b) fatty acids
   c) glucose
   d) protein

9. Bone, adipose tissue, epimysium, and hyaline cartilage are _____.
   a) areas of fat storage
   b) kinds of connective tissue
   c) skeletal structures
   d) common sites of inflammation

10. The thin tissue layer that forms the skin, organ coverings, and inner lining of all the hollow organs is the _____.
    a) epithelial tissue
    b) connective tissue
    c) muscular tissue
    d) skin

11. Fibrous tissue between muscle bundles is called _____.
    a) cartilage
    b) fascia
    c) muscular tissue
    d) perichondrium

12. The _____ membrane lines the inner joint cavities.   _____
    a) synovial   c) mucous
    b) adipose   d) serous

13. The bands that attach muscles to bone are _____.   _____
    a) tendons   c) cartilage
    b) ligaments   d) aponeuroses

14. The tough, fibrous bands that connect bones to bones are _____.   _____
    a) tendons   c) cartilage
    b) ligaments   d) fascia

15. Skeletal muscles are also known as _____.   _____
    a) voluntary muscles   c) tendinous muscles
    b) nonstriated muscles   d) smooth muscle

16. Cardiac muscle tissue occurs only in the _____.   _____
    a) liver   c) heart
    b) blood vessels   d) skeletal muscles

WORD REVIEW: Write down the meaning of each of the following words and titles. The list can be used later as a study guide for this chapter!

adipose tissue

_____

_____

_____

anabolism

_____

_____

_____

anaphase

_____

_____

_____

areolar tissue

_____

_____

_____

atoms

_____

_____

_____

cardiac muscle tissue

_____

_____

_____

catabolism

_____

_____

_____

cell

_____

_____

_____

cell membrane

_____

_____

_____

cellular metabolism

_____

_____

_____

centrosome

_____

_____

_____

columnar

_____

_____

_____

cuboidal

_____

_____

_____

cytoplasm

_____

_____

_____

cytoplasmic organelles

_____

_____

_____

dense connective tissue

_____

_____

_____

differentiation

_____

_____

_____

fibrocartilage

_____

_____

_____

enzymes

_____

_____

_____

epithelial membranes

_____

_____

_____

epithelial tissue

_____

_____

_____

fascia

_____

_____

_____

hyaline cartilage

_____

_____

_____

interphase

_____

_____

_____

ligaments

_____

_____

_____

metaphase

_____

_____

_____

mitosis

_____

_____

_____

molecules

_____

_____

_____

mucous membranes

_____

_____

_____

nerve tissue

_____

_____

_____

neurons

_____

_____

_____

nucleus

_____

_____

_____

organ system

_____

_____

_____

organs

_____

_____

_____

perichondrium

_____

_____

_____

periosteum

_____

_____

_____

prophase

_____

_____

_____

protoplasm

_____

_____

_____

reticular tissue

_____

_____

_____

serous membranes

_____

_____

_____

skeletal muscle

_____

_____

_____

smooth muscle

_____

_____

_____

squamous

_____

_____

_____

striated muscles

_____

_____

_____

superficial fascia

_____

_____

_____

synovial membrane

_____

_____

_____

telophase

_____

_____

_____

tendons

_____

_____

_____

tissues

_____

_____

_____

voluntary muscles

_____

_____

_____

THE ANATOMIC POSITION OF THE BODY

FILL-IN-THE-BLANK: In the space(s) provided, write the word(s) that correctly complete(s) each statement.

1. In the anatomic position, the body _____ with the palms of the hands facing _____ .

2. Anatomists divide the body with three imaginary planes called the _____ , the _____ , and the _____ planes.

3. The _____ divides the body into left and right parts by an imaginary line running vertically down the body.

4. The _____ is an imaginary line that divides the body into the anterior (front) or ventral half of the body and the posterior (back) or dorsal half of the body.

5. The _____ is an imaginary line that divides the body horizontally into an upper and lower portion.

6. _____ refers to the plane that divides the body or an organ into right and left halves.

MATCHING: Match the term with the best description. Write the letter of the best description in the space provided.

_____ 1. cranial or superior aspect

_____ 2. caudal or inferior aspect

_____ 3. anterior or ventral aspect

_____ 4. posterior or dorsal aspect

_____ 5. transverse plane

_____ 6. sagittal plane

_____ 7. coronal plane

_____ 8. medial aspect

_____ 9. lateral aspect

_____ 10. distal aspect

_____ 11. proximal

A. situated in front of

B. situated toward the tail

C. farthest point from the origin of a structure or point of attachment

D. situated in back of

E. on the side, farther from the midline

F. nearest the origin of a structure or point of attachment

G. situated toward the crown of the head

H. dividing the body into right and left sides

I. the frontal plane dividing it into front and back halves

J. pertaining to the middle or nearer to the midline

K. a plane through a body part perpendicular to the axis

IDENTIFICATION: Identify the indicated cavities in Figure 5-2 (a diagram of the various body cavities) by writing the correct names in the numbered space that corresponds to the number on the figure.

1. _____

2. _____

3. _____

4. _____

5. _____

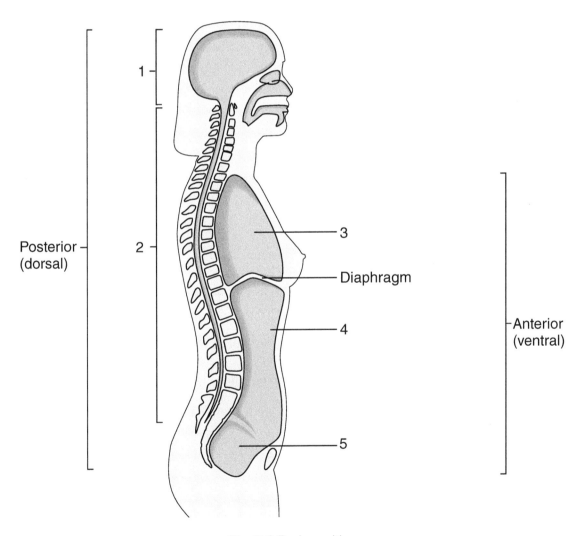

Fig. 5-2 Body cavities.

MATCHING: Match the term with the best description. Write the letter of the best description in the space provided.

_____ 1. hypogastric

_____ 2. inguinal

_____ 3. temporal

_____ 4. scapular

_____ 5. frontal

_____ 6. brachial

_____ 7. cervical

_____ 8. deltoid

_____ 9. umbilical

_____ 10. epigastric

_____ 11. lumbar

_____ 12. gluteal

_____ 13. patellar

_____ 14. popliteal

_____ 15. pectoral

_____ 16. parietal

_____ 17. axillary

_____ 18. femoral

_____ 19. mastoid

_____ 20. hypochondrium

A. region of the temples

B. region of the neck

C. region of the shoulder joint and deltoid muscle

D. region of the armpit

E. region between the elbow and the shoulder

F. region of the abdomen lateral to the epigastric region

G. region of the navel

H. region inferior to the umbilical region

I. region of the kneecap

J. region of the thigh

K. region of the groin

L. region of the lower back

M. region of the abdomen

N. region of the breast and chest

O. region of the head, posterior to the frontal region and anterior to the occipital region

P. region of the temporal bone behind the ear

Q. region of the muscles of the buttocks

R. region of the back of the shoulder or shoulder blade

S. an area behind the knee joint

T. region of the forehead

IDENTIFICATION: Identify the anatomic areas indicated in Figures 5-3 and 5-4 by writing the letter of the anatomic area next to the appropriate term in the space provided.

_____ 1. axillary   _____ 8. hypochondrium   _____ 15. pectoral

_____ 2. brachial   _____ 9. hypogastric   _____ 16. popliteal

_____ 3. cervical   _____ 10. inguinal   _____ 17. sacral

_____ 4. epigastric   _____ 11. lumbar   _____ 18. scapular

_____ 5. femoral   _____ 12. occipital   _____ 19. temporal

_____ 6. frontal   _____ 13. parietal   _____ 20. umbilical

_____ 7. gluteal   _____ 14. patellar

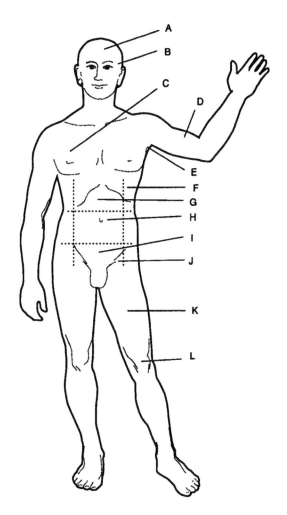

Fig. 5-3 Regions of the body, anterior view.

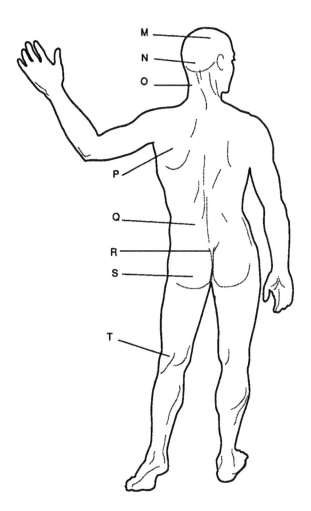

Fig. 5-4 Regions of the body, posterior view.

FILL-IN-THE-BLANK: In the space(s) provided, write the word(s) that correctly complete(s) each statement.

1. The dorsal cavities include the _____ cavity and the _____ cavity.

2. The ventral cavities are the _____ cavity and _____ cavity.

3. The liver, stomach, spleen, pancreas, and small and large intestines are located in the _____ cavity.

4. The _____ contains the bladder, rectum, and some of the reproductive organs.

5. The four main anatomic parts of the body are the _____, _____, _____, and _____.

6. Body structures containing two or more different tissues that combine to perform a definite function are called _____.

7. When several organs work together to perform a body function, they constitute an _____.

SHORT ANSWER: In the spaces provided, list 10 organ systems.

1. _____

2. _____

3. _____

4. _____

5. _____

6. _____

7. _____

8. _____

9. _____

10. _____

IDENTIFICATION: In the spaces provided, write the name of the related major body system.

_____ 1. carries oxygen and nutrients to all parts of the body

_____ 2. is damaged with a scratch or burn

_____ 3. provides a rigid structure and attachment for muscles

_____ 4. breaks down food into absorbable particles

_____ 5. includes the pituitary, thyroid, and ovaries

_____ 6. produces heat and movement

_____ 7. removes uric acid from the system

_____ 8. provides for continuation of the species

_____ 9. allows for the absorption of oxygen into the body

_____ 10. includes the kidneys, bladder, urethra, and ureters

_____ 11. provides information about where the body is in the environment

_____ 12. produces hormones

MULTIPLE CHOICE: Carefully read each statement. Choose the word or phrase that correctly completes the meaning and write the corresponding letter in the blank provided.

1. The imaginary line that divides the body into front and back halves is   _____
   the _____ plane.
   a) coronal   c) midsagittal
   b) sagittal   d) transverse

2. The liver and stomach are contained in the _____ cavity.   _____
   a) dorsal   c) abdominal
   b) pelvic   d) cranial

3. The elbow is _____ to the wrist.   _____
   a) proximal   c) lateral
   b) medial   d) distal

4. The ribs are lateral to the _____.   _____
   a) arms   c) pelvis
   b) scapula   d) sternum

5. Lumbar refers to the region of the _____.
   a) temple
   b) skull
   c) lower back
   d) pelvis

6. The epigastric area is _____.
   a) the location of the bladder
   b) inferior to the diaphragm
   c) the region of the tongue
   d) anterior to the scapula

7. The human body has _____ important organ systems.
   a) two
   b) five
   c) ten
   d) twenty

8. The axillary region of the body is _____.
   a) at the bend of the elbow
   b) the armpit
   c) near the groin
   d) on the head

9. The _____ region of the body is behind the knee.
   a) patellar
   b) parietal
   c) popliteal
   d) femoral

10. A sagittal cut through an organ or body divides it into _____.
    a) right and left portions
    b) superior and inferior portions
    c) dorsal and ventral portions
    d) three or four lateral portions

11. The bladder is located in the _____ cavity.
    a) dorsal
    b) cranial
    c) abdominal
    d) pelvic

12. A transverse section in the parietal area would show _____.
    a) the inside of the knee
    b) one side of the brain
    c) both sides of the brain
    d) both lungs

WORD REVIEW: Write down the meaning of each of the following words and titles. The list can be used later as a study guide for this chapter!

abdominal cavity

_____

_____

_____

anatomic position

_____

_____

_____

anterior

_____

_____

_____

circulatory system

_____

_____

_____

coronal plane

_____

_____

_____

cranial cavity

_____

_____

_____

digestive system

_____

_____

_____

distal

_____

_____

_____

dorsal cavities

_____

_____

_____

endocrine system

_____

_____

_____

caudal or inferior

_____

_____

_____

integumentary system

_____

_____

_____

lateral

_____

_____

_____

medial

_____

_____

_____

muscular system

_____

_____

_____

nervous system

_____

_____

_____

organ system

_____

_____

_____

pelvic cavity

_____

_____

_____

posterior

_____

_____

_____

proximal

_____

_____

_____

respiratory system

_____

_____

_____

sagittal plane

_____

_____

_____

skeletal system

_____

_____

_____

superior or cranial aspect

_____

_____

_____

thoracic cavity

_____

_____

_____

transverse plane

_____

_____

_____

urinary system

_____

_____

_____

ventral cavities

_____

_____

_____

vertebral or spinal cavity

_____

_____

_____

SYSTEM 1: REVIEW THE INTEGUMENTARY SYSTEM—THE SKIN

SHORT ANSWER: In the spaces provided, list six functions of the skin.

1. _____

2. _____

3. _____

4. _____

5. _____

6. _____

MATCHING: Match the term with the best description. Write the letter of the appropriate term in the space provided.

A. papillary layer   D. stratum corneum   G. dermis as a whole

B. reticular layer   E. stratum spinosum   H. epidermis as a whole

C. subcutaneous tissue   F. stratum germinativum

_____ 1. the deepest layer of the epidermis

_____ 2. contains fat cells, sweat and oil glands, and hair follicles

_____ 3. contains conelike projections made of fine strands of elastic tissue extending upward into the epidermis

_____ 4. site of keratin formation

_____ 5. contains blood and lymph vessels and nerve endings

_____ 6. serves as a protective cushion for the upper skin layers

_____ 7. contains melanocytes that produce the pigment melanin

_____ 8. contains collagen, reticulum, and elastin fibers

_____ 9. consists of cells containing melanin

IDENTIFICATION: Identify the structures indicated in Figure 5-5 (a cross-section of skin) by writing the letter of the structure next to the appropriate name in the space provided.

_____ 1. arrector pili muscle   _____ 3. epidermis

_____ 2. dermis   _____ 4. hair root

_____ 5. adipose

_____ 6. papilla of hair

_____ 7. capillaries

_____ 8. pacinian corpuscle

_____ 9. vein

_____ 10. hair shaft

_____ 11. Meissner corpuscle

_____ 12. reticular fibers

_____ 13. sebaceous gland

_____ 14. stratum corneum

_____ 15. stratum germinativum

_____ 16. stratum granulosum

_____ 17. subcutaneous tissue

_____ 18. dermal papilla

_____ 19. sudoriferous gland

_____ 20. stratum lucidum

_____ 21. stratum spinosum

_____ 22. artery

_____ 23. nerve

_____ 24. sweat pore

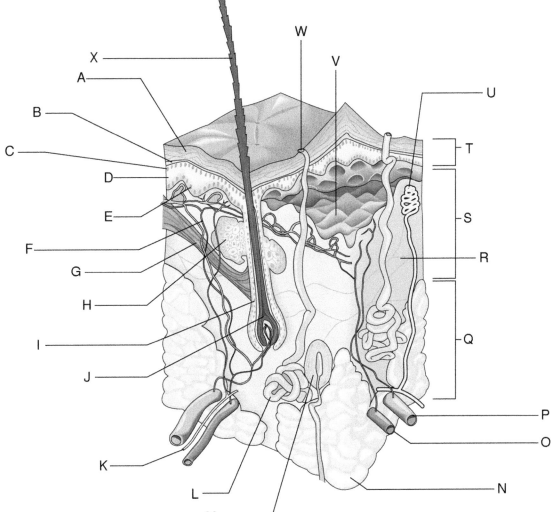

Fig. 5-5 The integumentary system (showing skin and hair).

TRUE OR FALSE: If the following statements are true, write *true* in the space provided. If they are false, replace the italicized word with one that makes the statement true.

_____ 1. There is a fine network of blood and lymph capillaries in the *epidermis*.

_____ 2. As people age, the *collagen* of the skin tends to lose its elasticity.

_____ 3. Pliability of the skin depends on the *sensory receptors* of the fibers in the dermis.

_____ 4. Healthy skin is soft, flexible, and slightly *acidic*.

_____ 5. The color of the skin depends on the *thickness* and the blood supply.

SHORT ANSWER: Circle the term that does not belong in each of the following groups (groups flow from left to right).

stratum germinativum	reticular layer	stratum malpighian	stratum granulosum
melanin	collagen	keratin	cuticle
pacinian corpuscle	ruffini corpuscle	arrector pili	Meissner corpuscle
scar	pustule	crust	fissure
seborrhea	leukoderma	lentigines	nevus

FILL-IN-THE-BLANK: In the space(s) provided, write the word(s) that correctly complete(s) each statement.

1. There are two clearly defined divisions of the skin. The outer layer is the _____ and the inner layer is the _____ .

2. There are two kinds of duct glands in the skin. _____ produce sweat and _____ glands produce oil.

3. Sweat glands are under the control of the _____ nervous system.

4. Two appendages of the skin are _____ and _____ .

5. The appendages of the skin referred to in the previous question are composed of _____ .

6. The _____ muscle is connected to the base of the hair follicle.

7. When the muscle referred to in the previous question contracts, it results in a reaction commonly called _____ .

8. A structural change in the tissues caused by injury or disease is a _____ .

9. A structural change in the tissues that develops in the later stages of disease is called

_____.

10. Small masses of hardened, discolored sebum that appear most frequently on the face, shoulders, chest, and back are called _____.

MATCHING: Match the term with the best description. Write the letter of the best description in the space provided.

_____ 1. scar

_____ 2. macule

_____ 3. pustule

_____ 4. scale

_____ 5. tumor

_____ 6. vesicle

_____ 7. bulla

_____ 8. ulcer

_____ 9. wheal

_____ 10. papule

_____ 11. crust

_____ 12. fissure

A. an accumulation of epidermal flakes

B. an itchy, swollen lesion that lasts only a few hours

C. an open lesion on the skin accompanied by loss of skin depth

D. a small, elevated pimple in the skin

E. a crack in the skin such as in chapped hands or lips

F. the scab on a sore

G. likely to form during the healing of an injury

H. an elevation of the skin having an inflamed base and containing pus

I. an external swelling, varying in size, shape, and color

J. a small, discolored spot or patch such as freckles

K. a blister similar to but larger than a vesicle

L. a blister with clear fluid in it

FILL-IN-THE-BLANK: In the space(s) provided, write the word(s) that correctly complete(s) each statement.

1. A skin inflammation caused by outside agents or chemicals is _____.

2. The most common type of skin cancer is _____

3. The most dangerous type of skin cancer is _____.

4. A mass of connected boils is a _____.

5. Three types of warts are _____, _____, and _____.

6. Three kinds of skin cancer are _____, _____, and _____.

7. The A-B-C-D-E signs for skin cancer are:

_____

_____

_____

_____

_____

8. _____ is a chronic, inflammatory skin condition characterized by round, dry patches covered with coarse, silvery scales.

9. _____ is a highly contagious, bacterial skin infection that is most common in children.

10. Another name for furuncle is _____ .

MULTIPLE CHOICE: Carefully read each statement. Choose the word or phrase that correctly completes the meaning and write the corresponding letter in the blank provided.

1. The largest organ of the body is the _____.   _____
   a) muscular system   c) liver
   b) skin   d) stomach

2. Protection, heat regulation, secretion, excretion, and absorption are   _____
   functions of the _____.
   a) endocrine system   c) muscles
   b) skin   d) brain

3. The deepest layer of the epidermis is the stratum _____.   _____
   a) germinativum   c) spinosum
   b) granulosum   d) lucidum

4. Collagen, reticulum, and elastin are the fibers in the cells of the   _____
   _____.
   a) epidermis   c) dermis
   b) lymph   d) blood

5. The skin gets its strength, form, and flexibility from _____.   _____
   a) collagen   c) the muscles
   b) elastin   d) subcutaneous tissue

6. A small discolored spot on the skin is a _____.
   a) macule   c) tumor
   b) bulla   d) vesicle

7. An elevation of the skin having an inflamed base and containing pus is a _____.
   a) papule   c) pustule
   b) pimple   d) wheal

8. A crack in the skin penetrating into the dermis is called a _____.
   a) fissure   c) scab
   b) crust   d) cut

9. Skin disorders are an area that massage therapists should be able to _____.
   a) treat successfully   c) recognize and refer
   b) use vibration on   d) apply antibiotic creams to

10. A generalized term for a structural change in tissue from disease or injury is _____.
    a) fracture   c) hematoma
    b) lesion   d) laceration

11. As epidermal cells at the base of a follicle are nourished, divide, die, and keratinize, they become _____.
    a) a shaft of hair   c) collagen fibers
    b) dermal cells   d) part of the epidermis

12. The subcutaneous layer consists of _____.
    a) epithelial tissue   c) loose connective tissue
    b) epithelium and loose connective tissue   and adipose tissue
                                                d) adipose tissue and
                                                   skeletal muscle tissue

13. A thickening in the skin caused by repeated or continued pressure is a _____.
    a) macule   c) bulla
    b) wheal   d) keratoma

14. An itchy swollen lesion that lasts only a few hours is a _____.
    a) tumor   c) bulla
    b) papule   d) wheal

15. Another name for skin is _____.
   a) cutaneous
   c) mucous
   b) integument
   d) serous

_____

16. "Goose bumps" are the result of _____.
   a) a nervous irritation
   c) body heat loss
   b) contracting arrector pili muscles
   d) oxygen depletion

_____

17. The _____ is a semi-solid part of the skin made up of a mixture of fibers, water, and "ground substance."
   a) endocrine
   c) dermis
   b) melanin
   d) epidermis

_____

18. The _____ comprises almost a solid sheet of cells at the outermost layers of the skin.
   a) dermis
   c) graft
   b) epidermis
   d) subcutaneous tissue

_____

19. When a body lies in one position too long, decreased circulation can result in _____, or "bedsores."
   a) decubitus ulcers
   c) acne rosacea
   b) apocrine
   d) hematomas

_____

WORD REVIEW: Write down the meaning of each of the following words and titles. The list can be used later as a study guide for this chapter!

collagen

_____

_____

_____

dermis

_____

_____

_____

epidermis

_____

_____

_____

integument

_____

_____

_____

keratin

_____

_____

_____

melanin

_____

_____

_____

reticular layer

_____

_____

_____

sebaceous gland

_____

_____

_____

stratum germinativum

_____

_____

_____

stratum granulosum

_____

_____

_____

stratum spinosum

_____

_____

_____

subcutaneous tissue

_____

_____

_____

sudoriferous gland

_____

_____

_____

SYSTEM 2: REVIEW THE SKELETAL SYSTEM

SHORT ANSWER: In the spaces provided, list the five main functions of the skeletal system.

1. _____

2. _____

3. _____

_____

4. _____

5. _____

KEY CHOICES: Bones are classified in one of four major bone forms or shapes. Put the appropriate key letter for each of the following bone classification in the space provided.

S = Short bones   I = Irregular bones

L = Long bones   F = Flat bones

_____ 1. tibia   _____ 7. axis

_____ 2. ilium   _____ 8. femur

_____ 3. phalange   _____ 9. talus

_____ 4. ulna   _____ 10. metacarpal

_____ 5. occiput   _____ 11. scapula

_____ 6. calcaneus   _____ 12. rib

FILL-IN-THE-BLANK: In the space(s) provided, write the word(s) that correctly complete(s) each statement.

1. The skeletal system is composed of _____, _____, and _____.

2. The inorganic mineral matter of bone consists mainly of _____ and _____ .

3. The fibrous membrane covering bone that serves as an attachment for tendons and ligaments is the _____.

4. The spongy bone tissue in flat bones and at the ends of long bones is filled with _____ and is the site of production for _____ .

5. The hollow chamber formed in the shaft of long bones that is filled with yellow bone marrow is the _____.

IDENTIFICATION: Identify the structures indicated in Figure 5-6 (a diagram of a typical long bone) by writing the correct letter in the space provided.

_____ 1. proximal epiphysis

_____ 2. compact bone

_____ 3. diaphysis (shaft of bone)

_____ 4. red marrow

_____ 5. distal epiphysis

_____ 6. medullary cavity (site of yellow bone marrow in adults)

_____ 7. periosteum (covering of bone)

_____ 8. spongy bone

_____ 9. articular cartilage

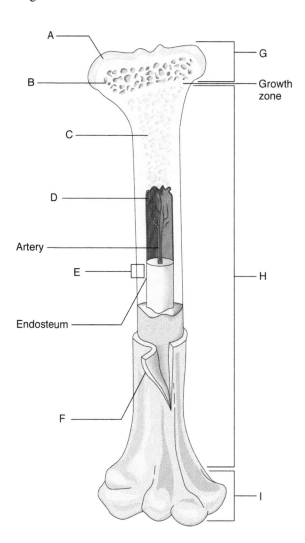

Fig. 5-6 Structure of a long bone.

FILL-IN-THE-BLANK: In the space(s) provided, write the word(s) that correctly complete(s) each statement.

1. The two main parts of the skeleton are the _____ and the _____.

2. The bones of the skull, thorax, vertebral column, and the hyoid bone make up the _____.

3. The bones of the shoulder, upper extremities, hips, and lower extremities make up the _____.

4. In the human adult, the skeleton consists of _____ bones.

5. The vertebral column consists of _____ bones.

6. There are _____ cervical vertebra.

7. There are _____ thoracic vertebra.

8. There are _____ lumbar vertebra.

9. There are _____ carpals in each wrist.

10. There are _____ tarsals in each ankle.

11. There are _____ phalanges in each hand.

12. The connection where two bones come together is called a _____ or an _____ .

13. The cranium is composed of _____ bones.

14. The face is composed of _____ bones.

KEY CHOICES: Joints are classified according to their structure and their function. In the first column of spaces provided, place the appropriate key letter indicating the structural classification next to the corresponding terms. In the second column, place the appropriate key letter indicating the functional classification next to the corresponding terms.

F = fibrous joints

C = cartilaginous joints

N = synovial joints

A = amphiarthrotic joints

D = diarthrotic joints

S = synarthrotic joints

Structural Classification

Functional Classification

1. symphysis pubis

2. glenohumeral joint

3. sagittal suture

4. elbow joint

5. bones united by fibrous connective tissue

6. hip joint

7. essentially immovable

8. sacroiliac joint

9. joint capsule with synovial fluid

10. intervertebral joints

11. articular cartilage on bones

12. joint between sphenoid and temporal bones

13. freely movable

14. allows limited movement

KEY CHOICE: Put the appropriate key letter for each of the following types of joints in the space provided. Movable joints in the body are classified descriptively

A. pivot joints

B. ball-and-socket joints

C. hinge joints

D. gliding joints

E.   saddle joints

F.   condyloid ellipsoid

G. symphysis

_____ 1. joint between ulna and humerus

_____ 2. hip joint

_____ 3. knee joint

_____ 4. joint between the first metacarpal and the trapezium

_____ 5. joints between radius and carpals

_____ 6. glenohumeral joint

_____ 7. joint between axis and atlas

_____ 8. joint between radius and ulna near elbow

_____ 9. intervertebral joints

_____ 10. interphalangeal joints

_____ 11. joint between the tibia and the talus

_____ 12. between right and left pubis

IDENTIFICATION: Identify the bones in Figure 5-7 by writing the correct label in the numbered space that corresponds to the number on the figure.

1. _____

2. _____

3. _____

4. _____

5. _____

6. _____

7. _____

8. _____

9. _____

10. _____

11. _____

12. _____

13. _____

14. _____

15. _____

16. _____

17. _____

18. _____

19. _____

20. _____

21. _____

22. _____

23. _____

24. _____

25. _____

26. _____

27. _____

28. _____

29. _____

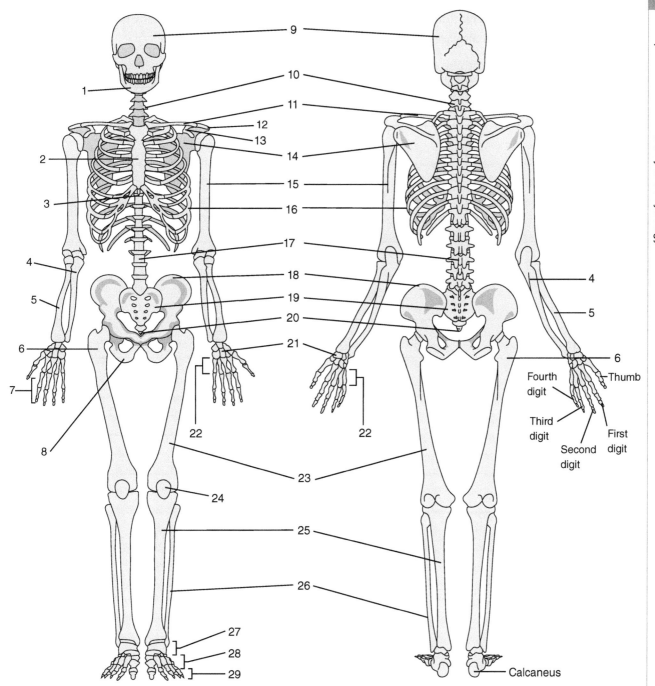

Fig. 5-7 Skeletal system, anterior view.

IDENTIFICATION: Identify the bony landmarks in Figures 5-8a and 5-8b by writing the correct name in the lettered space that corresponds to the letter in the figures.

A. _____

B. _____

C. _____

D. _____

   _____

E. _____

F. _____

G. _____

H. _____

I. _____

J. _____

K. _____

L. _____

M. _____

N. _____

O. _____

P. _____

Q. _____

R. _____

S. _____

T. _____

U. _____

V. _____

W. _____

X. _____

Y. _____

Z. _____

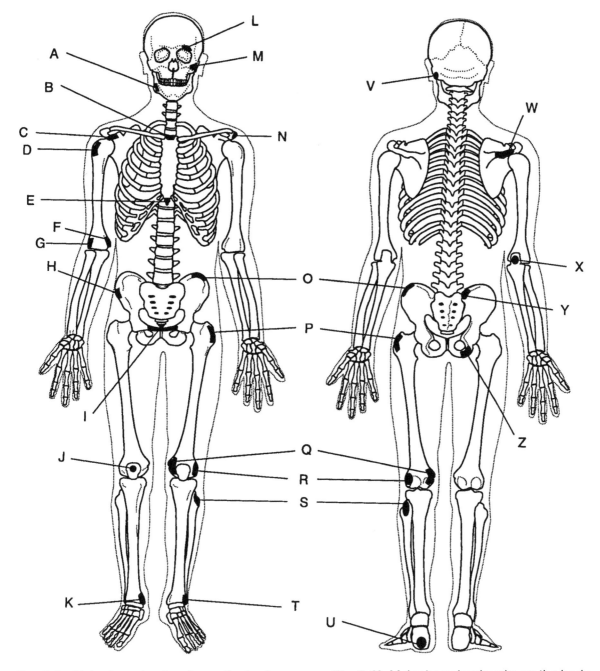

Fig. 5-8a Major bony landmarks on the body, anterior view.

Fig. 5-8b Major bony landmarks on the body, posterior view.

IDENTIFICATION: Identify the bones and sutures in Figure 5-9 by writing the number of the bone next to the appropriate term in the space provided.

_____ A. ethmoid   _____ F. nasal   _____ K. zygomatic arch

_____ B. frontal   _____ G. occipital   _____ L. coronal suture

_____ C. lacrimal   _____ H. parietal   _____ M. lambdoidal suture

_____ D. mandible   _____ I. sphenoid   _____ N. squamosal suture

_____ E. maxilla   _____ J. temporal

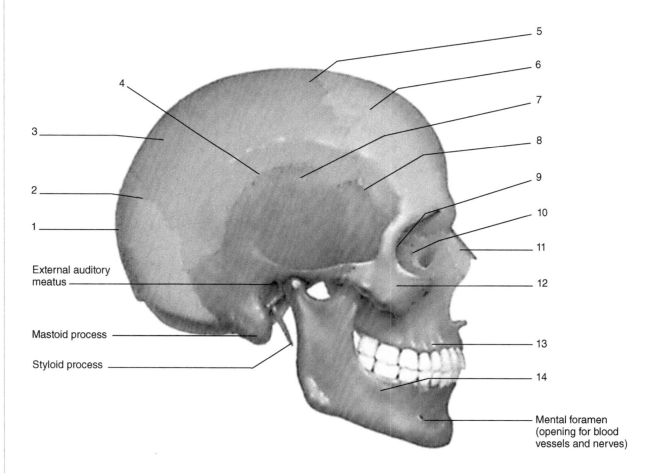

Fig. 5-9 Skeletal structures of the cranium, neck, and face.

IDENTIFICATION: Identify the parts of the spine in Figure 5-10 by writing the letter of the part next to the corresponding label in the space provided.

_____ 1. atlas, axis

_____ 2. cervical vertebrae

_____ 3. coccyx

_____ 4. lumbar vertebrae

_____ 5. sacrum

_____ 6. thoracic vertebrae

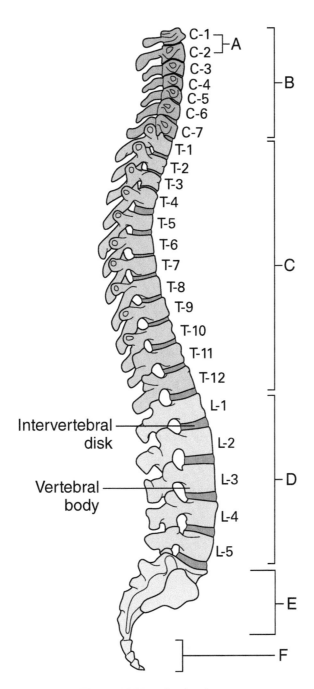

Fig. 5-10 Vertebral column.

MATCHING: Match the term with the best description. Write the letter of the best description in the space provided.

_____ 1. fossa   A. a less prominent ridge of a bone than a crest

_____ 2. trochanter   B. a rounded articulating process at the end of a bone

_____ 3. foramen   C. a large process for muscle attachment

_____ 4. sinus   D. a sharp slender projection

_____ 5. process   E. a tubelike passage

_____ 6. condyle   F. a depression or hollow

_____ 7. line   G. a ridge

_____ 8. tuberosity   H. a cavity within a bone

_____ 9. meatus   I. a rounded knuckle-like prominence usually at a point of articulation

_____ 10. tubercle

                                    J. a small rounded process

_____ 11. head

                                    K. a hole

_____ 12. spine

                                    L. a large rounded process

_____ 13. crest

                                    M. a bone prominence or projection

SHORT ANSWER: Circle the term that does not belong in each of the following groups (groups flow from left to right).

tibia	patella	femur	fibula
elbow	knee	finger	hip
axis/atlas	sacroiliac	intervertebral	pubic symphysis
tubercle	(fossa)	tuberosity	condyle
cranium	rib	vertebra	scapula

MATCHING: Match the skeletal disorders with the best description. Write the letter of the appropriate skeletal disorder in the space provided.

A. dislocation   C. osteoarthritis   E. fracture   G. bursitis

B. sprain   D. osteoporosis   F. rheumatoid arthritis

_____ 1. an inflammation of the small fluid-filled sacs located near the joints

_____ 2. a break or rupture in a bone

_____ 3. an inflammation causing the articular cartilage to erode and the joints to calcify and eventually become immovable

_____ 4. increased porosity of the bone that causes a thinning of bone tissue

_____ 5. displacement of a bone within a joint

_____ 6. a chronic inflammatory disease, that first affects the synovial membrane lining the joints

_____ 7. stretching or tearing of ligaments

_____ 8. a chronic disease that accompanies aging, usually affecting joints that have experienced a great deal of wear and tear or trauma

IDENTIFICATION: Identify each of the spinal curves in Figure 5-11 by writing the correct label in the space provided.

A. _____   B. _____   C. _____

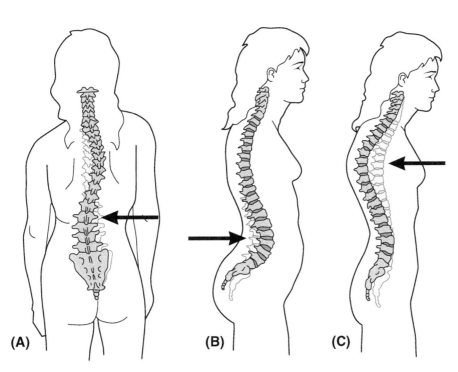

(A)   (B)   (C)

Fig. 5-11 Abnormal curvatures of the spine.

MULTIPLE CHOICE: Carefully read each statement. Choose the word or phrase that correctly completes the meaning and write the corresponding letter in the blank provided.

1. Flat bones are found in the _____.
   a) knee
   b) skull
   c) leg
   d) spine

   _____

2. The number of bones in the human adult skeleton is _____.
   a) 101
   b) 206
   c) 310
   d) 502

   _____

3. The bones of the upper and lower extremities form the _____.
   a) axial skeleton
   b) spine
   c) skull
   d) appendicular skeleton

   _____

4. White blood cells are produced by the _____.
   a) yellow bone marrow
   b) lymphocytes
   c) osteoclasts
   d) red bone marrow

   _____

5. A fracture in the shaft of the bone would be a break in the

   _____.
   a) epiphysis
   b) epiphyseal plate
   c) diaphysis
   d) articular cartilage

   _____

6. Muscle tendon fibers attach to bone by interlacing with _____.
   a) compact bone
   b) ligaments
   c) periosteum
   d) endosteum

   _____

7. Which of following is NOT a bone of the cranium?
   a) temporal
   b) sphenoid
   c) zygomatic
   d) parietal

   _____

8. The coracoid process is located _____.
   a) on the scapula
   b) behind the ear
   c) on the pelvis
   d) at the proximal end of
      the ulna

   _____

9. Immovable joints are called _____.
   a) amphiarthrotic
   b) articulations
   c) synarthrotic
   d) synovial

   _____

10. The range of motion of amphiarthrotic joints is _____.
    a) 360 degrees
    c) freely moving
    b) limited
    d) in a single plane

11. An example of a diarthrotic joint is _____.
    a) knee
    c) intervertebral
    b) skull
    d) the teeth

12. The greatest range of movement is found in _____.
    a) pivot joints
    c) ball-and-socket joints
    b) hinge joints
    d) saddle joints

13. A stretched ligament with some discomfort and minimal loss of
    function is a _____.
    a) Class I strain
    c) Class I sprain
    b) Class II sprain
    d) Class III sprain

14. The enlarged area on the end of long bones that articulates with
    other bones is called _____.
    a) the diaphysis
    c) articular cartilage
    b) the epiphysis
    d) cancellous tissue

15. Lateral curvature of the spine is called _____.
    a) lordosis
    c) convexity
    b) scoliosis
    d) kyphosis

16. Degenerative joint disease is generally known as _____.
    a) osteoporosis
    c) osteoarthritis
    b) rheumatoid arthritis
    d) osteomyelitis

17. Which of following is NOT a part of the pelvis?
    a) ischium
    c) zygomatic
    b) pubis
    d) ilium

18. The part of the long bone that is soft and contains the "growth line"
    is referred to as the _____.
    a) epiphysis
    c) bone shaft
    b) diaphysis
    d) bone marrow

19. The "ankle bone" that protrudes on the inside of the leg is the
    _____.

    a) medial malleolus   c) medial epicondyle

    b) fibula   d) lesser trochanter

                                      _____

20. The knee joint is an example of a _____ joint.

    a) synarthrotic   c) amphiarthrotic

    b) hinge   d) saddle

                                      _____

21. Which of the following is NOT found in the axial skeleton?

    a) the cranium   c) the sacrum

    b) the scapula   d) the sternum

                                      _____

22. The medial malleolus is on the _____.

    a) elbow   c) knee

    b) wrist   d) ankle

                                      _____

WORD REVIEW: Write down the meaning of each of the following words and titles. The list can be used later as a study guide for this chapter!

amphiarthrotic

_____

_____

_____

appendicular skeleton

_____

_____

_____

arthritis

_____

_____

_____

articular cartilage

_____

_____

_____

articulation

_____

_____

_____

axial skeleton

_____

_____

_____

bursae

_____

_____

_____

cartilage

_____

_____

_____

compact bone tissue

_____

_____

_____

cranium

_____

_____

_____

diaphysis

_____

_____

_____

diarthrotic joint

_____

_____

_____

epiphysis

_____

_____

_____

joint capsule

_____

_____

_____

kyphosis

_____

_____

_____

ligament

_____

_____

_____

lordosis

_____

_____

_____

marrow

_____

_____

_____

medullary cavity

_____

_____

_____

periosteum

_____

_____

_____

osteoporosis

_____

_____

_____

scoliosis

_____

_____

_____

sprain

_____

_____

_____

synarthrotic

_____

_____

_____

synovial fluid

_____

_____

_____

synovial membrane

_____

_____

_____

vertebra

_____

_____

_____

SYSTEM 3: REVIEW THE MUSCULAR SYSTEM

KEY CHOICES: There are three classifications of muscles. Put the appropriate key letter(s) for each of the following muscle types in the spaces provided.

A = skeletal   B = smooth   C = cardiac

_____ 1. contains striations

_____ 2. shapes and contours the body

_____ 3. forms the hollow organs

_____ 4. involved with transport of materials in the body

_____ 5. found only in the heart

_____ 6. spindle shaped

_____ 7. multinucleated

_____ 8. controlled by the autonomic nervous system

_____ 9. quadrangular in shape, joined end to end

_____ 10. contracts without direct nerve action

_____ 11. referred to as the muscular system

_____ 12. coordinates activity to act as a pump

FILL-IN-THE-BLANK: In the space(s) provided, write the word(s) that correctly complete(s) each statement.

1. The main tissue of the muscular system is _____.

2. Muscle cells have the unique ability to _____ .

3. Muscle comprises approximately_____ percent of a person's body weight.

4. The characteristics that enable muscles to perform their functions of contraction and movement are _____, _____, and _____.

5. The ability to return to its original shape after being stretched is _____ .

6. The capacity of muscles to receive and react to stimuli is _____ .

7. The ability to contract or shorten and thereby exert force is _____ .

STRUCTURE OF SKELETAL MUSCLES

FILL-IN-THE-BLANK: In the space(s) provided, write the word(s) that correctly complete(s) each statement.

1. The functional unit of a muscle is the _____ or _____.

2. The cell membrane of the muscle cell is the _____.

3. The connective tissue covering of the muscle cell is the _____.

4. Each muscle cell contains hundreds or even thousands of parallel _____.

5. The interaction of _____ and _____ filaments gives muscle its unique contractile ability.

6. The arrangement of _____ and _____ gives skeletal muscles a striated or striped appearance.

7. The site where the muscle fiber and nerve fiber meet is called the _____ or _____.

8. A motor neuron and all the muscle fibers that it controls constitute a _____.

9. When a nerve impulse reaches the end of the nerve fiber, a chemical neurotransmitter called _____ is released.

10. The energy for muscle contraction comes from the breakdown of the _____.

11. A metabolic process known as the _____ or the _____ takes place, resulting in the synthesis of ATP and the production of carbon dioxide, water, and energy in the form of heat.

12. When sufficient oxygen is available, ATP is synthesized through _____ respiration.

13. When the oxygen supply is depleted, ATP is synthesized through _____ respiration.

14. During strenuous activity, heavy breathing and accelerated heart rate are indications of _____.

15. Rapid or prolonged muscle contractions, to the point that oxygen debt becomes extreme and the muscle ceases to respond, causes _____.

16. The most stationary attachment of a muscle is the _____.

17. The muscle attachment that creates the action of the structure is the _____.

18. A(n) _____ contraction occurs when a muscle contracts and the ends of the muscle do not move.

19. The glistening cord that connects the muscle with its attachment is a _____.

IDENTIFICATION: Identify each skeletal muscle part in Figure 5-12 by writing the number of the part next to the appropriate term in the space provided.

_____ A. actin filament   _____ I. perimysium

_____ B. endomysium   _____ J. sarcolemma

_____ C. epimysium   _____ K. sarcoplasm

_____ D. fascicle   _____ L. tendon

_____ E. myofilament

_____ F. myofibril

_____ G. myosin filament

_____ H. muscle fiber

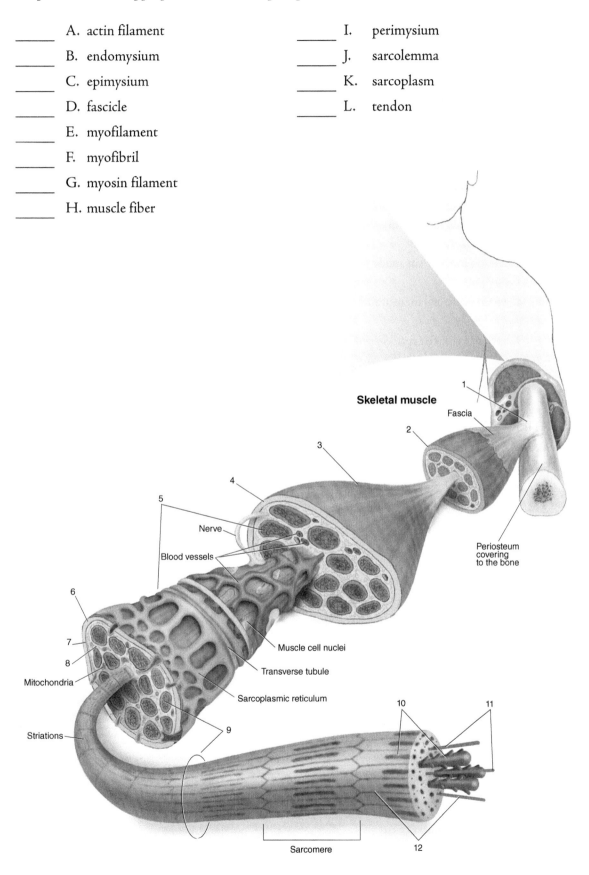

Fig. 5-12 Structure of skeletal muscle.

MATCHING: Match the skeletal muscle part listed above with the best description listed below. Write the letter of the skeletal muscle part in the space provided.

_____ 1. connective tissue projecting beyond the end of the muscle

_____ 2. connective tissue covering the entire muscle

_____ 3. separates muscles into bundles of fibers

_____ 4. connective tissue covering of each muscle cell

_____ 5. bundle of muscle fibers

_____ 6. contractile unit of muscle tissue

_____ 7. a protein filament made up of actin

_____ 8. the muscle cell membrane

_____ 9. structure of the muscle cell containing actin and myosin

_____ 10. the muscle cell intercellular fluid

IDENTIFICATION: Identify each part of the muscle cell sarcomere in Figure 5-13 by writing the appropriate letter next to the correct term in the space provided.

_____ 1. A band

_____ 2. actin filament

_____ 3. H zone

_____ 4. I band

_____ 5. M line

_____ 6. myosin filament

_____ 7. sarcomere

_____ 8. Z line

_____ 9. zone of overlap

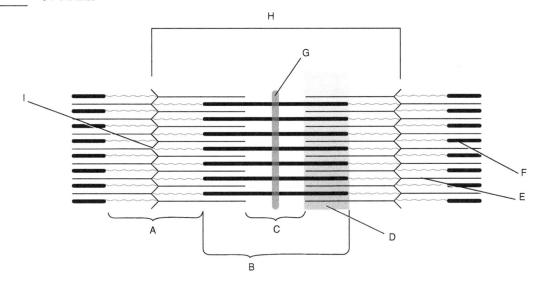

Fig. 5-13 Parts of the muscle cell.

MATCHING: Match the term with the best description. Write the letter of the appropriate term in the space provided.

    A. Type I muscle fibers   B. Type II muscle fibers

_____ 1. able to sustain low-level muscle contractions

_____ 2. darker red color

_____ 3. depend on anaerobic metabolism

_____ 4. fast twitch fibers

_____ 5. fatigue easily

_____ 6. have fewer mitochondria

_____ 7. high capacity to generate ATP

_____ 8. high resistance to fatigue

_____ 9. high number of mitochondria

_____ 10. larger fibers with more actin and myosin filaments

_____ 11. lighter color

_____ 12. more prominent in phasic muscles

_____ 13. more prominent in postural muscles

_____ 14. produce powerful, fast contractions

_____ 15. rich capillary supply

_____ 16. slow twitch fibers

_____ 17. tend to tighten and shorten when stressed

_____ 18. uses aerobic metabolism

_____ 19. vulnerable to muscle strains and tendonitis

IDENTIFICATION: On the following list of muscles, identify the postural muscles by placing a "P" in the space provided.

_____ 1. adductor longus and magnus   _____ 3. deltoid

_____ 2. anterior neck flexors   _____ 4. gluteals

_____ 5. iliopsoas

_____ 6. latissimus dorsi

_____ 7. levator scapulae

_____ 8. lower pectorals

_____ 9. lumbar erector spinae

_____ 10. middle and lower trapezius

_____ 11. oblique abdominals

_____ 12. pectoralis minor

_____ 13. peroneals

_____ 14. piriformis

_____ 15. quadratus lumborum

_____ 16. rectus abdominis

_____ 17. rectus femoris

_____ 18. rhomboids

_____ 19. sacrospinalis

_____ 20. scalenii

_____ 21. serratus anterior

_____ 22. sternocleidomastoid

_____ 23. tensor fascia lata

_____ 24. triceps

_____ 25. upper trapezius

_____ 26. vastus muscles

TRUE OR FALSE: If the following statements are true, write _true_ in the space provided. If they are false, replace the italicized word with one that makes the statement true.

_____ 1. Muscle fibers are attached to bone by connective tissue called _ligaments_.

_____ 2. Each motor nerve attaches to _one_ muscle cell.

_____ 3. The release of calcium ions by the sarcoplasmic reticulum results in a _muscle contraction_.

_____ 4. A skeletal muscle by definition has _both ends_ attached to bone.

_____ 5. Only enough ATP is stored in muscle to sustain a muscle contraction for a few _minutes_.

_____ 6. ATP is produced by the _mitochondria_.

_____ 7. An eccentric contraction is an _isotonic_ contraction.

FILL-IN-THE-BLANK: In the space(s) provided, write the word(s) that correctly complete(s) each statement.

1. A(n) _____ contraction occurs when a muscle is contracted and the ends of the muscle move further apart.

2. A(n) _____ contraction occurs when a muscle is contracted and the ends of the muscle move closer together.

3. Eccentric and concentric muscle contractions are both _____ contractions.

4. When an action occurs, the muscle that is responsible for that action is the _____ .

5. When an action occurs, the muscle that is responsible for the opposite action is the _____ .

6. Muscles that assist the primary muscle of an action are called _____ .

7. When discussing the dynamics of the movement of the body, the three components of motion are _____ , _____ , and _____ .

MATCHING: Match the term with the best description. Write the letter of the best description in the space provided.

_____ 1. posterior	A. that which presses or draws down
_____ 2. dilator	B. behind or in back of
_____ 3. inferior	C. pertaining to the middle or center
_____ 4. oblique	D. before or in front of
_____ 5. levator	E. situated lower
_____ 6. dorsal	F. to straighten
_____ 7. superior	G. that which lifts
_____ 8. medial	H. behind or in back of
_____ 9. distal	I. nearer to the center or medial line
_____ 10. depressor	J. at an angle
_____ 11. proximal	K. farther from the center or medial line
_____ 12. anterior	L. situated above
_____ 13. extensor	M. that which expands or enlarges

MATCHING: Match the term with the best description. Write the letter of the appropriate term in the space provided.

_____ 1. raise the shoulders toward the ears

_____ 2. action of the neck when looking at the ceiling

_____ 3. action of the hip when standing up out of a seated position

_____ 4. action of the toes when standing on tiptoes

_____ 5. turning the hand palm up

_____ 6. action of the foot when pointing toes

_____ 7. action of elbow during eccentric contraction of bicep

_____ 8. bringing the knees together

_____ 9. action of knee during concentric contraction of biceps femoris

_____ 10. turning the sole of the foot medially

_____ 11. action of the femur when turning the feet outward

_____ 12. action of the hip when bringing the knee toward the chest

_____ 13. turning the palm of the hand downward

_____ 14. action of the foot when pointing the toes up toward the knee

A. flexion

B. extension

C. dorsiflexion

D. plantar flexion

E. adduction

F. abduction

G. pronation

H. supination

I. medial rotation

J. lateral rotation

K. circumduction

L. hyperextension

M. inversion

N. eversion

O. elevation

P. depression

FILL-IN-THE-BLANK: In the space(s) provided, write the word(s) that correctly complete(s) each statement.

1. A sudden involuntary contraction of a muscle or a group of muscles is a

    _____.

2. An enlargement of the breadth of a muscle as a result of repeated forceful muscle activity is called _____.

3. When the muscle tissue degenerates and begins to waste away, the process is called

    _____.

4. A group of related diseases that seems to be genetically inherited and that causes a progressive degeneration of the voluntary muscular system is _____.

5. _____ is characterized by pain, fatigue, and stiffness in the connective tissue of the muscles, tendons, and ligaments. It is associated with stress and poor sleep habits and is most prevalent in women.

6. An inflammation of the tendon often occurring at the musculotendinous junction is

    _____.

7. An inflammation of the tendon sheath that is often accompanied by pain and swelling is called

    _____.

SHORT ANSWER: Circle the term that does not belong in each of the following groups (groups flow from left to right).

brachioradialis	biceps brachii	brachialis	coracobrachialis
biceps femoris	rectus femoris	vastus medialis	vastus lateralis
supraspinatus	subscapularis	teres major	teres minor
pectineus	rectus femoris	adductor longus	gracilis
teres major	pectoralis major	subscapularis	infraspinatus

IDENTIFICATION: Identify the muscles in Figure 5-14 by writing the correct name in the numbered space that corresponds to the number in the figure.

The Muscular System—Anterior View

1. _____

2. _____

3. _____

4. _____

5. _____

6. _____

7. _____

8. _____

9. _____

10. _____

11. _____

12. _____

13. _____

14. _____

15. _____

16. _____

17. _____

18. _____

19. _____

20. _____

21. _____

22. _____

23. _____

24. _____

25. _____

26. _____

27. _____

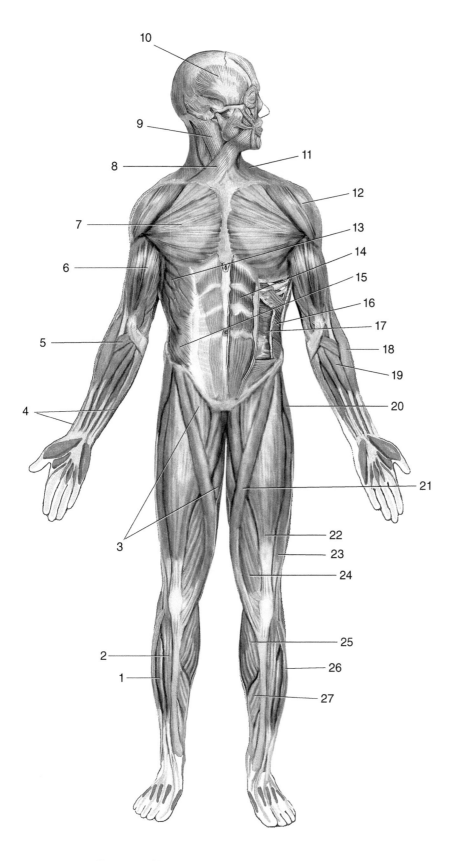

Fig. 5-14 The muscular system, anterior view.

IDENTIFICATION: Identify the muscles in Figure 5-15 by writing the correct name in the numbered space that corresponds to the number in the figure.

The Muscular System—Posterior View

1. _____

2. _____

3. _____

4. _____

5. _____

6. _____

7. _____

8. _____

9. _____

10. _____

11. _____

12. _____

13. _____

14. _____

15. _____

16. _____

17. _____

18. _____

19. _____

20. _____

21. _____

22. _____

23. _____

24. _____

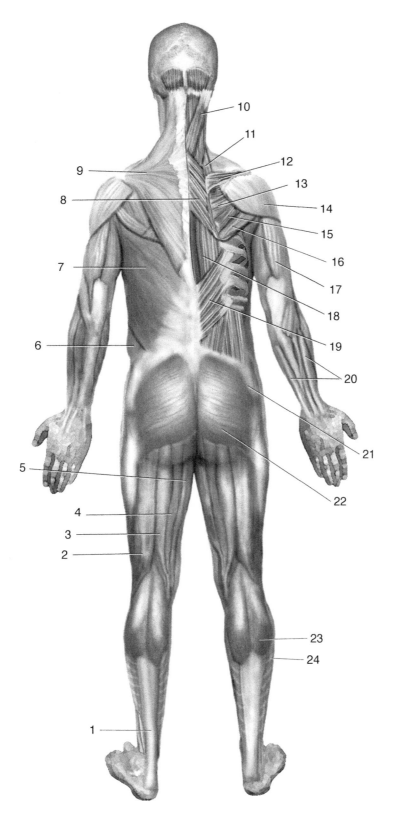

Fig. 5-15 The muscular system, posterior view.

MATCHING: In the first answer column, identify the body part the muscle acts on. Write the correct letter in the answer blank. In the second answer column, indicate the action the muscle causes when it contracts. Write the correct letter in the answer blank.

Body part   **Action**

_____   _____   1. gluteus medius   A. Flexes

_____   _____   2. triceps brachii   B. Extends

_____   _____   3. upper trapezius   C. Adducts

_____   _____   4. deltoid (medial)   D. Abducts

_____   _____   5. gastrocnemius   E. Elevates

_____   _____   6. gluteus maximus   F. Plantar flexes

_____   _____   7. adductor magnus   G. Dorsal flexes

_____   _____   8. latissimus dorsi   H. Big toe

_____   _____   9. biceps femoris   I. Elbow

_____   _____   10. tibialis anterior   J. Thumb

_____   _____   11. peroneus longus   K. Hip

_____   _____   12. gracilis   L. Ankle

_____   _____   13. rectus femoris   M. Knee

_____   _____   14. vastus lateralis   N. Scapula

_____   _____   15. biceps brachii   O. Wrist

_____   _____   16. pectoralis major   P. Neck

_____   _____   17. sternocleidomastoid   Q. Shoulder

_____   _____   18. palmaris longus   R. Finger

_____   _____   19. Sartorius

_____   _____   20. tensor fascia lata

_____   _____   21. abductor pollicis longus

_____   _____   22. extensor hallucis longus

_____   _____   23. brachioradialis

_____   _____   24. extensor indicis

_____   _____   25. soleus

_____   _____   26. iliopsoas

_____   _____   27. supraspinatus

MULTIPLE CHOICE: Carefully read each statement. Choose the word or phrase that correctly completes the meaning and write the corresponding letter in the blank provided.

1. The ability of muscle to return to its original shape after being stretched is called _____. _____
   - a) contractility
   - b) resizing
   - c) elasticity
   - d) shortening

2. The layer of connective tissue that covers an individual muscle is called the _____. _____
   - a) fascicle
   - b) epimysium
   - c) periosteum
   - d) endomysium

3. Each muscle fiber within a fascicle is covered by tissue called _____. _____
   - a) epimysium
   - b) periosteum
   - c) endomysium
   - d) perimysium

4. Muscle's contractile ability is a result of the interaction between two filaments, myosin and _____. _____
   - a) actin
   - b) elastin
   - c) adenosine
   - d) reticulin

5. Which type of muscle tissue is found in the heart wall? _____
   - a) nonstriated
   - b) cardiac
   - c) smooth
   - d) skeletal

6. The cell membrane of a muscle fiber is called the _____. _____
   - a) endomysium
   - b) sarcolemma
   - c) sarcoplasmic reticulum
   - d) fascia

7. The striated appearance of skeletal muscles results from the _____. _____
   - a) sarcoplasmic reticulum network
   - b) transverse tubule pattern
   - c) sarcomere arrangement
   - d) aerobic conversion

8. The strength of a muscle contraction is varied by changing the _____. _____
   - a) number of motor units stimulated
   - b) strength that each individual fiber contracts
   - c) number of fibers contracting within each motor unit
   - d) the intensity of the nerve impulse

9. The transmission of the stimulus of muscle contraction is aided by
   _____ .
   a) myosin   c) brain waves
   b) actin   d) transverse tubules

10. Energy for muscle contractions comes from _____ .
    a) ATF   c) ADP
    b) CPA   d) ATP

11. _____ is found in the gap between the end of the motor nerve
    and the muscle fiber.
    a) Mitochondria   c) Acetylcholine
    b) Adenosine triphosphate   d) Creatine phosphate

12. The condition in which muscles cease to respond because of lack of
    oxygen and/or buildup of waste products is called _____ .
    a) muscle fatigue   c) lactic acid
    b) oxygen deficiency   d) anaerobic respiration

13. A muscle contraction in which the body part affected by the muscle
    does not move is called _____ .
    a) isotonic   c) eccentric
    b) isometric   d) concentric

14. A muscle contraction in which the distance between the ends of the
    muscle changes is called _____ .
    a) isotonic   c) dynamic
    b) resistant   d) isometric

15. The muscle that originates on the coracoid process and flexes the
    elbow is the _____ .
    a) brachioradialis   c) biceps brachii
    b) brachialis   d) coracobrachialis

16. A muscle that flexes the neck or turns the head to the opposite side is
    the _____ .
    a) splenius capitus   c) sternocleidomastoid
    b) scalenus posterior   d) all of the above

17. A muscle strain that involves a partial tear of 10-50 percent of the
    muscle fibers is classified _____.   _____
    a) Grade I   c) Grade III
    b) Grade II   d) parietal

18. A group of related genetic diseases that cause progressive
    degeneration of the voluntary muscular system is called _____.   _____
    a) muscular dystrophy   c) fibrosis
    b) myofibrosis   d) atrophy

19. Aerobic cellular respiration to replenish ATP takes place in the   _____

    _____.
    a) liver   c) mitochondria
    b) bloodstream   d) cell nucleus

WORD REVIEW: Write down the meaning of each of the following words and titles. The list can
be used later as a study guide for this chapter!

abduction

_____

_____

_____

actin

_____

_____

_____

adduction

_____

_____

_____

antagonist

_____

_____

_____

aponeurosis

_____

_____

_____

cardiac muscle

_____

_____

_____

contractility

_____

_____

_____

elasticity

_____

_____

_____

extensibility

_____

_____

_____

extension

_____

_____

_____

fascia

_____

_____

_____

flexion

_____

_____

_____

insertion

_____

_____

_____

motor neuron

_____

_____

_____

motor unit

_____

_____

_____

muscle fatigue

_____

_____

_____

myofibril

_____

_____

_____

myosin

_____

_____

_____

origin

_____

_____

_____

oxygen debt

_____

_____

_____

prime mover

_____

_____

_____

pronation

_____

_____

skeletal muscle

_____

_____

smooth muscle

_____

_____

striated

_____

_____

supination

_____

_____

synergist

_____

_____

tendon

_____

_____

SYSTEM 4: REVIEW THE CIRCULATORY SYSTEM

FILL-IN-THE-BLANK: In the space(s) provided, write the word(s) that correctly complete(s) each statement.

1. The two divisions to the vascular system are the _____ _____ and _____.

2. The double-layered membrane that covers the heart is the _____.

3. The normal heart rate for an adult is _____ beats per minute.

4. The blood vessels that carry blood away from the heart are the _____ and _____.

5. The blood vessels that carry blood back toward the heart are the _____ and _____

6. The largest artery in the body is the _____ .

7. The smallest, microscopic, thin-walled blood vessels are called _____.

8. The two circulation systems in the blood-vascular system are _____ and _____.

TRUE OR FALSE: If the following statements are true, write *true* in the space provided. If they are false, replace the italicized word with one that makes the statement true.

_____ 1. Impulses from the sympathetic portion of the autonomic nervous system cause *vasodilation*.

_____ 2. Substances move through the capillary walls mostly by *osmosis*.

_____ 3. Blood moves through the *arterioles* to the capillaries and then to the *venules*.

_____ 4. *Diffusion* is a process in which substances move from an area of higher pressure to lower pressure.

_____ 5. In *pulmonary* circulation, veins contain oxygen-rich blood.

IDENTIFICATION: Identify the parts indicated in Figure 5-16 (a cross-section of a portion of the heart wall, including the pericardium) by writing the letter of the part next to the appropriate term in the space provided.

_____ 1. epicardium

_____ 2. myocardium

_____ 3. endocardium

_____ 4. parietal pericardium

_____ 5. pericardial cavity

_____ 6. visceral pericardium

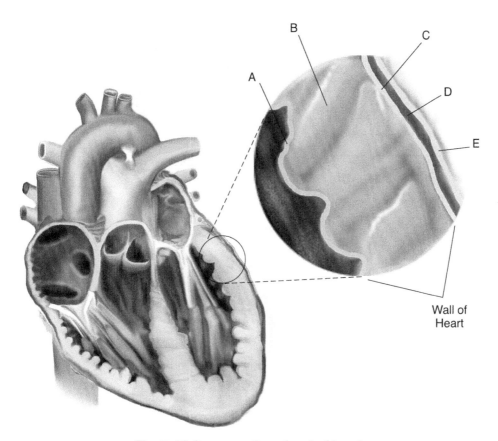

Fig. 5-16 Cross-section of wall of heart.

TRUE OR FALSE: If the following statements are true, write _true_ in the space provided. If they are false, replace the italicized word with one that makes the statement true.

_____ 1. The cardiovascular system of the average adult male contains about _eleven_ pints of blood.

_____ 2. Blood has a slightly _acid_ reaction.

_____ 3. Plasma accounts for 75 percent of the blood's volume.

_____ 4. _White blood cells_ constitute as much as 98 percent of all blood cells.

_____ 5. Red blood cells and _white blood cells_ are produced in the red bone marrow

IDENTIFICATION: Identify the structures of the heart indicated in Figure 5-17 (a diagram of the frontal structure of the heart) by writing the letter next to the appropriate term in the space provided.

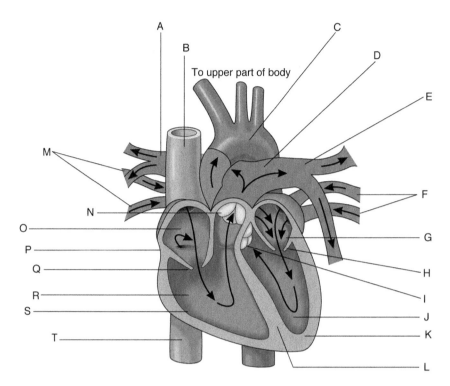

Fig. 5-17 Frontal section of the heart.

_____ 1. aorta

_____ 2. aortic semilunar valve

_____ 3. inferior vena cava

_____ 4. left atrium

_____ 5. left ventricle

_____ 6. mitral (bicuspid) valve

_____ 7. left pulmonary artery

_____ 8. pulmonary semilunar valve

_____ 9. pulmonary veins

_____ 10. right atrium

_____ 11. right ventricle

_____ 12. septum

_____ 13. superior vena cava

_____ 14. tricuspid valve

_____ 15. right pulmonary artery

_____ 16. endocardium

_____ 17. pericardium

_____ 18. pulmonary trunk

_____ 19. myocardium

MATCHING: Match the term with the best description. Write the letter of the appropriate term in the space provided.

A. arteriosclerosis   C. embolus   E. atherosclerosis

B. phlebitis   D. varicose veins   F. edema

_____ 1. protruding, bulbous, distended superficial veins

_____ 2. an inflammation of a vein

_____ 3. a condition of excess fluid in the interstitial spaces

_____ 4. the walls of affected arteries tend to thicken, become fibrous, and lose their elasticity

_____ 5. an accumulation of fatty deposits on the inner walls of the arteries

_____ 6. a clot that breaks loose and floats in the bloodstream

SHORT ANSWER: Five functions of the blood are listed below. In the spaces provided, briefly describe how the blood performs these functions.

1. Blood provides nutrients to the cells.

_____

_____

_____

2. Blood removes wastes.

_____

_____

_____

3. Blood maintains normal body temperature.

_____

_____

_____

4. Blood protects against infection.

_____

_____

_____

5. Blood prevents hemorrhaging.

_____

_____

_____

FILL-IN-THE-BLANK: In the space(s) provided, write the word(s) that correctly complete(s) each statement.

1. Red blood cells are also called _____.

2. Red blood cells are colored with an oxygen-carrying substance called _____.

3. The process in which leukocytes actually engulf and digest harmful bacteria is called

   _____.

4. The small irregularly shaped particles in the blood that play an important role in clotting are
   _____ or _____ .

5. A disease characterized by extremely slow clotting of blood and excessive bleeding from even
   very slight cuts is _____.

6. A condition in which there is a rapid loss or inadequate production of red blood cells is

   _____

7. A form of cancer in which there is an uncontrolled production of white blood cells is known as

   _____.

TRUE OR FALSE: If the following statements are true, write *true* in the space provided. If they are false, replace the italicized word with one that makes the statement true.

_____ 1. Lymph is derived from the interstitial fluid and is *produced* by the lymph nodes.

_____ 2. Lymphoid tissue produces a kind of white blood cell called a *lymphocyte*.

_____ 3. All lymph eventually flows into the bloodstream.

_____ 4. The right lymphatic duct collects lymph from the *right half of the body*.

_____ 5. Lymph is moved through the lymph system by a pumping action of the *lymph nodes*.

FILL-IN-THE-BLANK: In the space(s) provided, write the word(s) that correctly complete(s) each statement.

1. Specialized white blood cells called _____ play a major role in the immune response.

2. White blood cells originate in _____.

3. White blood cells specialize into T-cells in the _____.

4. The agent that triggers an immune response is a(n) _____.

5. White blood cells are transported throughout the body by _____ and
_____.

6. The production of antibodies is the responsibility of the _____.

7. When the immune system mistakenly attacks itself, the result is _____.

8. _____ attack and destroy antigens directly.

9. The cell that is destroyed by the HIV virus in AIDS is the _____ .

10. When is an HIV infected person considered to have AIDS?

_____

_____

11. How is HIV transmitted from one person to another?

_____

_____

12. The process of specialized cells engulfing and digesting neutralized antigens and debris is
_____.

SHORT ANSWER: Circle the term that does not belong in the following groups (groups flow from left to right).

spleen	liver	tonsils	thymus
lacteal	thoracic duct	lymphatic	venule
swelling	nausea	pain	redness
lymphocytes	monocytes	platelets	leukocytes
lymph capillaries	capillary beds	closed system	continuous flow

IDENTIFICATION: Identify the numbered blood vessels in Figure 5-18 (a diagram of the major blood vessels of the body) by writing the correct term in the numbered space that corresponds to the number on the figure. (The arteries are indicated on the left side of the body as unshaded vessels. The veins are indicated on the right side of the body as shaded vessels.)

1. _____

2. _____

3. _____

4. _____

5. _____

6. _____

7. _____

8. _____

9. _____

10. _____

11. _____

12. _____

13. _____

14. _____

15. _____

16. _____

17. _____

18. _____

19. _____

20. _____

21. _____

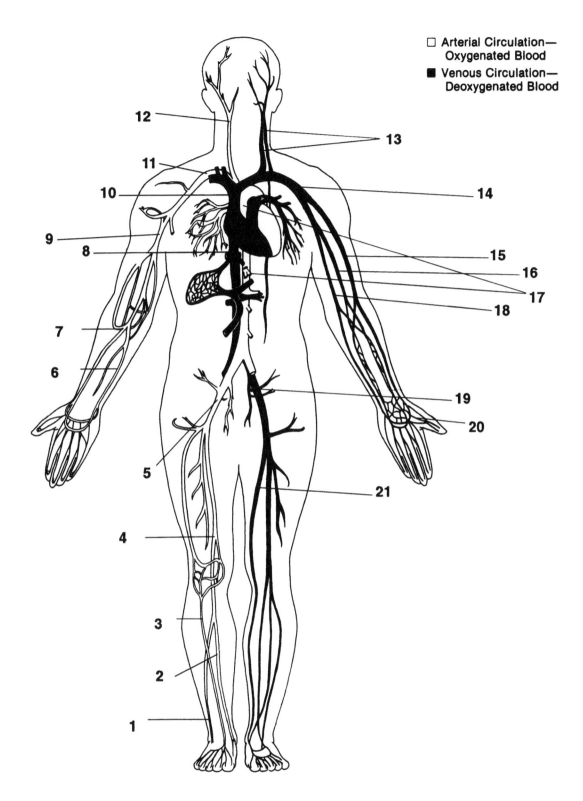

□ Arterial Circulation—
Oxygenated Blood
■ Venous Circulation—
Deoxygenated Blood

Fig. 5-18 Circulatory system.

MATCHING: Match the terms with the best description. Write the letter of the appropriate term in the space provided.

A. acquired immunity   D. memory cells   G. innate immunity

B. immunity   E. vaccines   H. autoimmune diseases

C. allergen   F. allergy

_____ 1. stimulate an immune response without causing the accompanying illness

_____ 2. all the physiologic mechanisms used by the body as protection against foreign substances

_____ 3. is present from before birth

_____ 4. allergy-causing substance

_____ 5. specialized form of immunity that is the result of an encounter with a new substance

_____ 6. overreaction by the immune system to an otherwise harmless substance

_____ 7. when the body makes antibodies and T-cells directed against its own cells

_____ 8. provide immunity for years or even a lifetime

TRUE OR FALSE: If the following statements are true, write *true* in the space provided. If they are false, replace the italicized word with one that makes the statement true.

_____ 1. Acquired immunodeficiency syndrome (*AIDS*) disease occurs when the human immunodeficiency virus (HIV) enters a person's body.

_____ 2. An HIV-infected person is clinically said to have AIDS when their CD4 + T-cell blood count falls below *500* per cubic millimeter of blood.

_____ 3. HIV is spread most commonly by *sexual contact* with an infected partner or through contact with infected blood.

_____ 4. Massage *is* contraindicated for people infected with HIV or AIDS.

_____ 5. Health care workers can reduce their risk of becoming HIV infected in their practice by following *safe sex* precautions.

MULTIPLE CHOICE: Carefully read each statement. Choose the word or phrase that correctly completes the meaning and write the corresponding letter in the blank provided.

1. Supplying the body with nutrients and carrying away waste products is the function of the _____.
   a) lungs
   b) circulatory system
   c) kidneys
   d) muscles

2. The two-way diffusion of substances between the blood and tissue fluids surrounding cells is the function of the _____.
   a) arteries
   b) veins
   c) capillaries
   d) lymph

3. Waste-laden blood returns to the heart through the _____.
   a) veins
   b) arteries
   c) capillaries
   d) lymphatics

4. Blood platelets are important to proper _____.
   a) nutrition
   b) clotting
   c) immunity
   d) circulation

5. Macrophages are large cells that destroy foreign bacteria by the process of _____.
   a) osmosis
   b) mitosis
   c) phagocytosis
   d) enzymatic action

6. The process in which substances move from an area of higher concentration to an area of lower concentration is _____.
   a) diffusion
   b) osmosis
   c) filtration
   d) saturation

7. Blood is supplied to the small finger side of the hand by the _____.
   a) ulnar artery
   b) popliteal artery
   c) parietal artery
   d) radial artery

8. The right atrium receives blood directly from _____.
   a) the superior and inferior vena cava
   b) the right ventricle
   c) the pulmonary veins
   d) the coronary vein

9. The liquid that surrounds tissue cells is called _____.
   a) lymph
   b) interstitial fluid
   c) plasma
   d) blood

10. Toxic substances and harmful bacteria are filtered by the _____.
    a) lymphatic system
    b) spleen
    c) muscular system
    d) bone marrow

11. Lymph reenters the blood-vascular system through the _____.
    a) lymph capillaries
    b) lymph nodes
    c) spleen
    d) subclavian vein

12. Approximately how much of the fluid that leaves the blood-vascular system is absorbed by the lymph-vascular system?
    a) 5 percent
    b) 10 percent
    c) 20 percent
    d) 40 percent

13. A condition in which there is an inadequate population of red blood cells is _____.
    a) hemophilia
    b) anemia
    c) edema
    d) leukemia

14. Blood from the face and cranium is drained by the _____.
    a) external jugular vein
    b) subclavian vein
    c) inferior vena cava
    d) cephalic veins

15. The inside membrane lining the heart and the valves is called _____.
    a) the endocardium
    b) the myocardium
    c) the pericardium
    d) the epicardium

16. The pulmonary semilunar valve prevents the backflow of blood into _____.
    a) the lung
    b) the right atrium
    c) the right ventricle
    d) the left atrium

17. An erythrocyte _____.
    a) manufactures antibodies
    b) releases serotonin
    c) contains hemoglobin
    d) performs phagocytosis

18. Which of the following are white blood cells? _____
   a) leukocytes
   b) mononeuritis
   c) hemoglobin
   d) all of the above

19. A free-floating blood clot is called _____. _____
   a) an embolism
   b) thrombosis
   c) phlebitis
   d) an embolus

WORD REVIEW: Write down the meaning of each of the following words. The list can be used as a study guide for this chapter!

anemia

_____

_____

_____

aorta

_____

_____

_____

arteriole

_____

_____

_____

arteriosclerosis

_____

_____

_____

artery

_____

_____

_____

atrium

_____

_____

_____

auricle

_____

_____

_____

blood-vascular system

_____

_____

_____

capillary

_____

_____

_____

cardiovascular system

_____

_____

_____

diffusion

_____

_____

_____

edema

_____

_____

_____

embolus

_____

_____

_____

endocardium

_____

_____

_____

epicardium

_____

_____

_____

erythrocytes

_____

_____

_____

filtration

_____

_____

_____

hemoglobin

_____

_____

_____

interstitial

_____

_____

_____

lacteal

_____

_____

_____

leukemia

_____

_____

_____

leukocytes

_____

_____

_____

lymph

_____

_____

_____

lymph-vascular system

_____

_____

_____

lymphatic pump

_____

_____

_____

lymphatics

_____

_____

_____

mitral valve

_____

_____

_____

myocardium

_____

_____

_____

pericardial cavity

_____

_____

_____

pericardium

_____

_____

_____

phagocytosis

_____

_____

_____

phlebitis

_____

_____

_____

plasma

_____

_____

_____

platelets

_____

_____

_____

pulmonary circulation

_____

_____

_____

semilunar valve

_____

_____

_____

systemic circulation

_____

_____

_____

thoracic duct

_____

_____

_____

thrombocytes

_____

_____

_____

tricuspid valve

_____

_____

_____

vasoconstriction

_____

_____

_____

vasodilation

_____

_____

_____

vasomotor nerves

_____

_____

_____

vein

_____

_____

_____

vena cava

_____

_____

_____

ventricle

_____

_____

_____

venules

_____

_____

_____

SYSTEM 5: REVIEW THE NERVOUS SYSTEM

FILL-IN-THE-BLANK: In the space(s) provided, write the word(s) that correctly complete(s) each statement.

1. The major parts of the nervous system are the _____, _____ , and _____.

2. The structural unit of the nervous system is the _____ or _____.

3. There are two types of nerve fibers. _____ connect with other neurons to receive information and a single _____ conducts impulses away from the cell body.

4. Impulses are passed from one neuron to another at a junction called a _____.

5. Two characteristics of a neuron are _____ and _____.

6. Neurons that originate in the periphery and carry information toward the central nervous system (CNS) are _____ or _____ neurons.

7. Neurons that carry impulses from the brain to the muscles or glands that they control are _____ or _____ neurons.

8. Neurons located in the brain and spinal cord that carry impulses from one neuron to another are _____.

9. The portion of the nervous system that is surrounded by bone is the _____, which consists of the _____ and the _____.

10. The CNS is covered by a special connective tissue membrane called the _____, which has three layers: _____, the _____, and the _____.

11. The fluid that surrounds and supports the brain and spinal cord is _____.

12. The largest portion making up the front and top of the brain is the _____.

13. The smaller part of the brain that helps to maintain the body's balance and coordinates voluntary muscles is the _____.

14. The three parts of the brain stem are the _____, the _____, and the _____.

15. The two divisions of the peripheral nervous system are the _____, which involves the nerves to the visceral organs, glands, and blood vessels, and the _____, which involves the nerves to the muscles and skin.

IDENTIFICATION: Identify the structures indicated in Figure 5-19 (a diagram of a nerve cell) by writing the letter of the structure next to the correct term in the space provided.

_____ 1. axon

_____ 2. cell body

_____ 3. dendrites

_____ 4. myelin sheath

_____ 5. nucleus

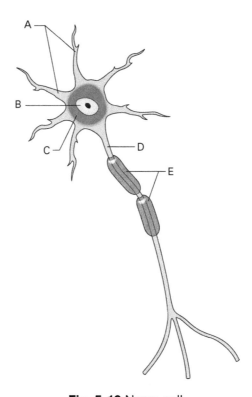

Fig. 5-19 Nerve cell.

MATCHING: Match the term with the best description. Write the letter of the appropriate term in the space provided.

A. afferent neuron

B. axon

C. dendrite

D. efferent neuron

E. interneuron

F. nerve

G. stimuli

H. synapse

_____ 1. the conducting portion of a neuron

_____ 2. junction point between neurons

_____ 3. bundle of nerve fibers in the peripheral nervous system

_____ 5. changes that activate the nervous system

_____ 6. receptive structure of the neuron

_____ 7. carries sensory information to the brain

_____ 8. transmits information from one neuron to another

TRUE OR FALSE: If the following statements are true, write *true* in the space provided. If they are false, replace the italicized word with one that makes the statement true.

_____ 1. The spinal cord extends from the medulla oblongata to the *sacrum*.

_____ 2. Control centers in the *pons* regulate movements of the heart and control vasoconstriction of the arteries.

_____ 3. The *midbrain* relays impulses from the cerebrum to the cerebellum.

_____ 4. Spinal nerves are numbered according to *the level where they exit the spine*.

_____ 5. There are *thirty-one* pairs of spinal nerves.

_____ 6. All of the nerves outside the brain and spinal cord are considered to be the *peripheral* nervous system.

CRANIAL NERVES

IDENTIFICATION AND MATCHING: Number the cranial nerves according to the order in which they arise from the brain. In the first column of answer blanks, write the Roman numeral that corresponds to the cranial nerve. Then, select the best description of the function of the cranial nerve from the list below the table, and write the appropriate letter in the second column of answer blanks.

Number   Function

_____ _____   1. trochlear nerve   A. shoulder; movement of neck muscles

_____ _____   2. optic nerve   B. sensations of the face and movement of the jaw and tongue

_____ _____   3. hypoglossal nerve   C. moves eyeball down and out

_____ _____   4. vagus nerve   D. sensation and movement related to talking, heart rate, breathing, and digestion

_____ _____   5. spinal accessory nerve

_____ _____   6. abducens nerve   E. sense of smell

_____ _____   7. oculomotor nerve   F. moves eyeball up, down, and in; constricts pupil; raises eyelid

_____ _____   8. trigeminal nerve   G. tongue movement

_____ _____   9. auditory nerve   H. movements of the face and some muscles of the neck and ear

_____ _____   10. olfactory nerve   I. moves eyeball outward

_____ _____   11. glossopharyngeal nerve   J. sense of taste

_____ _____   12. facial nerve   K. sense of sight

                                                      L. sense of hearing

SHORT ANSWER: In the spaces provided, write the answers to the following questions.

1. How many pairs of cervical nerves are there? _____

2. How many pairs of thoracic nerves are there? _____

3. How many pairs of lumbar nerves are there? _____

4. How many pairs of sacral nerves are there? _____

MATCHING: Match the term with the best description. Write the letter of the appropriate term in the space provided.

A. mechanoreceptors   C. photoreceptors   E. nociceptors

B. thermoreceptors   D. chemoreceptors

_____ 1. detect heat or cold

_____ 2. detect color

_____ 3. detect pain

_____ 4. proprioceptors

_____ 5. respond to tissue damage and extreme stimuli

_____ 6. Ruffini end organs and Merkel disks

_____ 7. rods and cones in the retina

_____ 8. sense pressure, vibration

_____ 9. sense smell and taste

IDENTIFICATION: Identify the major parts of the nervous system in Figure 5-20 by writing the letter of the part next to the appropriate term in the space provided.

_____ 1. autonomic chain of ganglia   _____ 6. intercostal nerve

_____ 2. brachial plexus   _____ 7. lumbar plexus

_____ 3. brain   _____ 8. median nerve

_____ 4. cervical plexus   _____ 9. plantar nerve

_____ 5. femoral nerve   _____ 10. peroneal nerve

_____ 11. radial nerve

_____ 12. sacral plexus

_____ 13. saphenous nerve

_____ 14. sciatic nerve

_____ 15. spinal cord

_____ 16. tibial nerve

_____ 17. ulnar nerve

_____ 18. spinal nerve

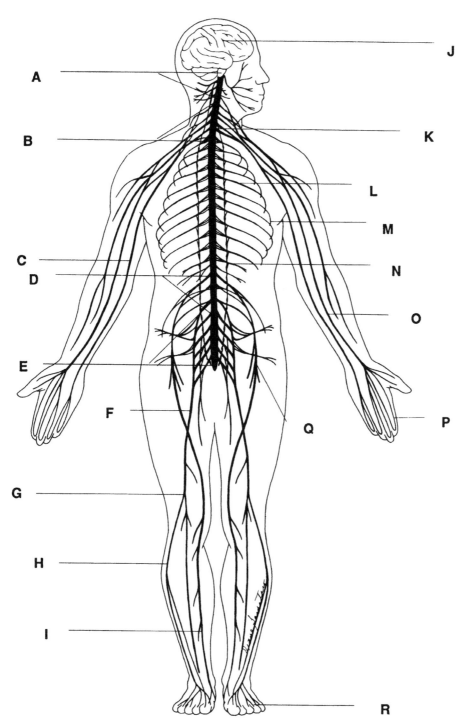

Fig. 5-20 The nervous system.

MATCHING: Match the term with the best description. Write the letter of the term in the space provided.

A. central nervous system   D. autonomic nervous system

B. peripheral nervous system   E. sympathetic nervous system

C. somatic nervous system   F. parasympathetic nervous system

_____ 1. Stimulation causes increased respiration, dilated pupils, increased heart rate, and cardiac output.

_____ 2. Consists of cranial nerves, spinal nerves and all their branches.

_____ 3. Is completely housed and protected in a bony covering.

_____ 4. General function is to conserve energy.

_____ 5. Is composed of the sympathetic and parasympathetic nervous system.

_____ 6. Includes the autonomic and somatic nervous system.

_____ 7. Nerve fibers arise from the second, third, and fourth sacral spinal nerves and the III, VII, IX, and X (vagus nerve) cranial nerves.

_____ 8. Is composed of the brain and spinal cord.

_____ 9. Prepares the organism for energy-expending, stressful, or emergency situations.

_____ 10. Regulates smooth muscle, the heart, and other involuntary functions.

_____ 11. Interprets incoming information and issues orders.

_____ 12. Carries information to and from all parts of the body.

_____ 13. Carries information to and from the skeletal muscles and skin.

_____ 14. Involves a chain of ganglia located along the spine.

FILL-IN-THE-BLANK: In the space(s) provided, write the word(s) that correctly complete(s) each statement.

1. The simplest form of nervous activity that includes a sensory and motor nerve and few, if any, interneurons is called a _____ .

2. The nerve pathway of the simplest form of nervous activity is called a _____ .

IDENTIFICATION: Identify the structures indicated in Figure 5-21 (a diagram of a simple reflex arc) by writing the letter of the structure next to the appropriate term in the space provided. (Note the arrows that indicate the direction of the nerve impulse.)

_____ 1. sensory neuron

_____ 2. dorsal root

_____ 3. motor neuron

_____ 4. connecting neuron

_____ 5. sensory nerve receptor

_____ 6. spinal cord

_____ 7. spinal ganglion

_____ 8. ventral root

_____ 9. muscle (effector)

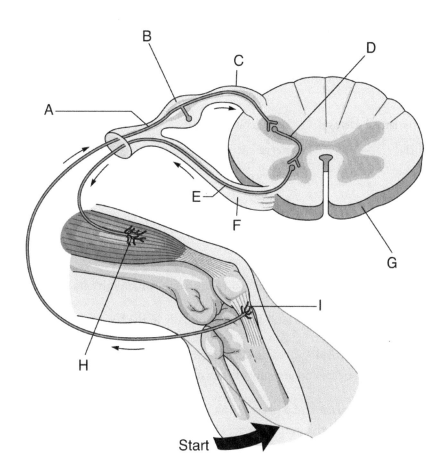

Fig. 5-21 Simple reflex arc.

FILL-IN-THE-BLANK: In the space(s) provided, write the word(s) that correctly complete(s) each statement.

1. Sensory nerves that record conscious sensations such as heat, cold, pain, and pressure are termed _____.

2. Sensory nerves that respond to the unconscious inner sense of position and movement of the body are termed _____.

3. The system of sensory and motor nerve activity that provides information as to the position and rate of movement of different body parts is _____.

4. _____ sense the length and stretch of the muscle as well as how far and fast the muscle is moving.

5. _____ consist of intrafusal muscle fibers, annulospiral, and flower-type nerve receptors.

6. _____ are multibranched sensory nerve endings located in tendons in the area where muscle fibers attach to tendon tissue.

7. _____ measure the amount of tension produced in muscle cells that occur as a result of the muscle's stretching and contracting.

MATCHING: Match the term with the best description. Write the letter of the appropriate term in the space provided.

A. amyotrophic lateral sclerosis G. nerve compression   L. poliomyelitis

B. encephalitis   H. nerve entrapment   M. quadriplegia

C. epilepsy   I. neuritis   N. shingles

D. hemiplegia   J. paraplegia   O. spinal cord injury

E. meningitis   K. Parkinson's disease   P. stroke

F. multiple sclerosis

_____ 1. the result of the breakdown of the myelin sheath, which inhibits nerve conduction

_____ 2. characterized by tremors and shaking, especially in the hands

_____ 3. a degenerative neurologic condition affecting the motor nerves of the brain, causing weakness, spasticity, and atrophy of the voluntary muscles

_____ 4. an acute inflammation of a nerve trunk and the dendrites at the end of the sensory neurons, caused by the herpes zoster virus

_____ 5. paralysis of the lower part of the body

_____ 6. paralysis affecting the arms and the legs

_____ 7. paralysis affecting one side of the body

_____ 8. the inflammation of a nerve that is usually a symptom of some other condition

_____ 9. the result of a blood clot or ruptured blood vessel in or around the brain

_____ 10. abnormal electrical activity in the CNS characterized by seizures

_____ 11. caused by soft tissue, such as muscle, fascia, tendon, or ligament, that puts pressure against a nerve

_____ 12. a crippling or even deadly disease that affects the motor neurons of the medulla oblongata and spinal cord, resulting in paralysis

_____ 13. caused by disease or trauma to the vertebral column, resulting in loss of sensation and movement to the body below the site of injury

_____ 14. a viral disease causing inflammation of the brain and meninges

_____ 15. an acute inflammation of the pia and arachnoid mater around the brain and spinal cord

_____ 16. caused by bone or cartilage pressing against the nerve

MULTIPLE CHOICE: Carefully read each statement. Choose the word or phrase that correctly completes the meaning and write the corresponding letter in the blank provided.

1. The junction at which impulses are passed from one neuron to another is called a/an _____.   _____
   a) axon   c) synapse
   b) neuromuscular junction   d) dendrite

2. The central nervous system consists of the spinal cord and the _____.   _____
   a) motor neurons   c) mixed nerves
   b) afferent nerves   d) brain

3. A motor neuron is also called a/an _____.   _____
   a) efferent neuron   c) nerve cell
   b) interneuron   d) afferent neuron

4. The three types of neurons are _____.   _____
   a) sympathetic, parasympathetic, peripheral
   b) afferent, efferent, connecting
   c) sensory, motor, interneuron
   d) receptors, effectors, conductors

5. Body balance and voluntary muscle movement are controlled by the
   _____.
   a) cerebellum
   c) brain stem
   b) cerebrum
   d) midbrain

6. The spinal cord has _____ pairs of spinal nerves.
   a) 25
   c) 42
   b) 31
   d) 36

7. Movement of head, neck, and shoulders is controlled by the
   _____.
   a) cervical plexus
   c) brachial plexus
   b) somatic system
   d) cranial nerves

8. All thought, speech, memories, and emotion take place in the
   _____.
   a) cerebrum
   c) cerebral cortex
   b) thalamus
   d) medulla oblongata

9. The largest and longest nerve in the body is the _____ nerve.
   a) brachial
   c) lumbar
   b) vagus
   d) sciatic

10. Damage to the _____ nerve could cause inability of the diaphragm
    to function.
    a) phrenic
    c) hypoglossal
    b) axillary
    d) pneumogastric

11. Specialized nerve endings that sense the amount of tension produced
    in muscle cells are called _____.
    a) spindle cells
    c) exteroceptors
    b) Golgi tendon organs
    d) Ruffini end organs

12. Which of the following are considered peripheral nerves?
    a) cranial nerves
    c) sympathetic nerves
    b) spinal nerves
    d) all of the above

13. The parasympathetic and sympathetic nervous systems constitute the
    _____.
    a) central nervous system
    c) autonomic nervous system
    b) peripheral nervous system
    d) none of the above

14. The axon is a nerve fiber _____.
    a) carrying the impulse toward the cell body
    b) that is the body's communication center
    c) carrying the impulse away from the cell body
    d) with sensory function only

15. Annulospiral receptors and Golgi tendon organs are parts of the

    _____.

    a) proprioceptors   c) exteroceptors
    b)autonomic nervous system   d) central nervous system

16. The three brain coverings are collectively known as the _____.
    a) thalamus   c) meninges
    b) motor cortex   d) convolutions

17. The pons, midbrain, and medulla oblongata form the _____.
    a) cerebral hemispheres   c) brain stem
    b) cerebellum   d) cerebral cortex

18. _____ serves as the insulating sheath covering the axon.
    a) cerebrospinal fluid   c) pia mater
    b) myelin   d) meninges

19. A condition in which there is an inflammation of one or more
    peripheral nerves is _____.
    a) meningitis   c) neuralgia
    b) neuritis   d) encephalitis

20. Often a stroke causes a type of paralysis called _____.
    a) cerebrovascular accident   c) quadriplegia
    b) paraplegia   d) hemiplegia

WORD REVIEW: Write down the meaning of each of the following words. The list can be used as a study guide for this chapter!

afferent nerve

_____

_____

_____

afferent neuron

_____

_____

_____

arachnoid mater

_____

_____

_____

autonomic nervous system

_____

_____

_____

axon

_____

_____

_____

brachial plexus

_____

_____

_____

brain

_____

_____

_____

brain stem

_____

_____

_____

central nervous system

_____

_____

_____

cerebellum

_____

_____

_____

cerebrospinal fluid

_____

_____

_____

cerebrovascular accident

_____

_____

_____

cerebrum

_____

_____

_____

cervical plexus

_____

_____

_____

cranial nerves

_____

_____

_____

dendrite

_____

_____

_____

dura mater

_____

_____

_____

efferent nerve

_____

_____

_____

efferent neuron

_____

_____

_____

epilepsy

_____

_____

_____

ganglia

_____

_____

_____

Golgi tendon organs

_____

_____

_____

hemiplegia

_____

_____

_____

interneuron

_____

_____

_____

kinesthesia

_____

_____

_____

lumbar plexus

_____

_____

_____

medulla oblongata

_____

_____

_____

meninges

_____

_____

_____

mixed nerve

_____

_____

_____

motor nerve

_____

_____

_____

motor neuron

_____

_____

_____

muscle spindle cells

_____

_____

_____

nerve

_____

_____

_____

nerve cell

_____

_____

_____

nerve fibers

_____

_____

_____

neuralgia

_____

_____

_____

neuritis

_____

_____

_____

neuron

_____

_____

_____

neurotransmitter

_____

_____

_____

paraplegia

_____

_____

_____

parasympathetic nervous system

_____

_____

_____

peripheral nervous system

_____

_____

_____

pia mater

_____

_____

_____

pons

_____

_____

_____

proprioception

_____

_____

_____

proprioceptors

_____

_____

_____

quadriplegia

_____

_____

_____

reflex

_____

_____

_____

reflex arc

_____

_____

_____

sacral plexus

_____

_____

_____

sciatic nerve

_____

_____

_____

sciatica

_____

_____

_____

sensory nerve

_____

_____

_____

sensory neuron

_____

_____

_____

somatic nervous system

_____

_____

_____

spinal cord

_____

_____

_____

spinal cord injury

_____

_____

_____

stroke

_____

_____

_____

sympathetic nervous system

_____

_____

_____

synapse

_____

_____

_____

SYSTEM 6: REVIEW THE ENDOCRINE SYSTEM

FILL-IN-THE-BLANK: In the space(s) provided, write the word(s) that correctly complete(s) each statement.

1. Glands that have tubes or ducts that carry their secretions to a particular part of the body are
   _____ or _____.

2. Glands that depend on the blood and lymph to carry their secretions to various affected tissues
   are _____ glands.

3. The chemical substances manufactured by the endocrine glands are known as
   _____.

IDENTIFICATION: Identify the hormone-producing organs in Figure 5-22 by writing the correct term in the numbered space that corresponds to the number on the figure. Also name the hormone-producing organs described in numbers 10, 11, and 12.

A.

1. _____   6. _____

2. _____   7. _____

3. _____   8. _____

4. _____   9. _____

5. _____

B.

_____ 10. The posterior and anterior pituitaries hang from the bottom of this hormone-producing organ.

_____ 11. This is present only in pregnant women.

_____ 12. These are the four small glands attached to the thyroid.

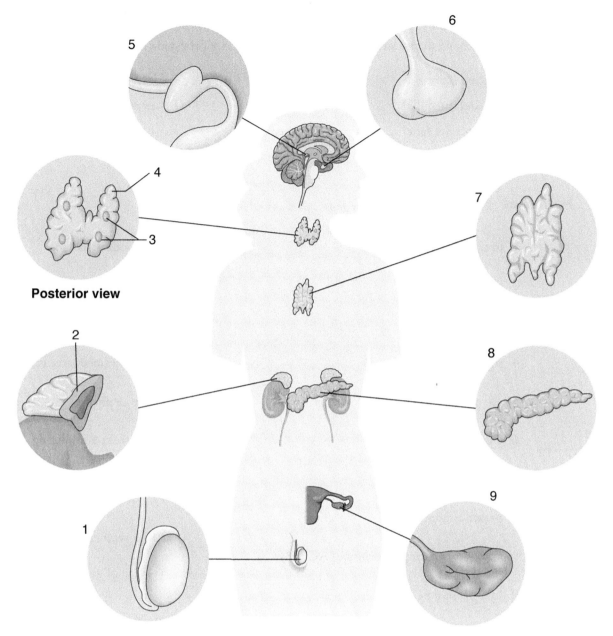

Posterior view

Fig. 5-22 The endocrine system.

MATCHING: Using the following list of organs, match the organ with the hormone(s) that it produces or releases. Write the letter of the organ(s) in the space provided.

A. adrenal gland (cortex)

B. adrenal gland (medulla)

C. pituitary (anterior lobe)

D. pituitary (posterior lobe)

E. ovaries

F. testes

G. pancreas

H. thymus

I. thyroid

J. parathyroid

K. pineal

Hormones

_____ 1. prolactin

_____ 2. aldosterone

_____ 3. insulin

_____ 4. thyroxin

_____ 5. estrogen

_____ 6. Cortisol

_____ 7. calcitonin

_____ 8. parathormone

_____ 9. adrenocorticotropic hormone (ACTH)

_____ 10. hydrocortisone

_____ 11. gonadotropic hormones

_____ 12. glucagon

_____ 13. triiodothyronine

_____ 14. oxytocin

_____ 15. progesterone

_____ 16. mineralocorticoids

_____ 17. epinephrine

_____ 18. thyroid-stimulating hormone (TSH)

_____ 19. testosterone

_____ 20. norepinephrine

_____ 21. growth hormone

_____ 22. corticosteroids

_____ 23. antidiuretic hormone

MATCHING: Match the term with the best description. Write the letter of the appropriate term in the space provided.

A. adrenocorticotropic

B. aldosterone

C. calcitonin

D. Cortisol

E. estrogen

F. follicle-stimulating hormone

G. glucagon

H. insulin

I. lactogenic hormone

J. luteinizing hormone

K. oxytocin

L. parathormone

M. progesterone

N. TSH

_____ 1. antagonistic to insulin, produced by the same gland

_____ 2. promotes the lining of the uterus to thicken in preparation for fertilization

_____ 3. anterior pituitary hormones that stimulates hormone activity of ovarian follicles

_____ 4. stimulates development of secretory parts of mammary glands

_____ 5. directly regulate the menstrual cycle

_____ 6. stimulates thyroid to produce thyroxin

_____ 7. decreases calcium in the blood

_____ 8. increases calcium level in the blood

_____ 9. stimulates mammary glands to secrete milk

_____ 10. helps protect the body during stress; stimulates the adrenal cortex

_____ 11. necessary for glucose to be taken up by cells

IDENTIFICATION: The following list of conditions are usually the result of hyper- or hypoactivity of an endocrine gland's production of a particular hormone. In the first answer column, indicate whether the condition is caused by to hyper- or hypoactivity. In the second answer column, write the name of the hormone involved.

Activity   **Hormone**

_____   _____   1. giantism

_____   _____   2. Addison's disease

_____   _____   3. Graves disease

_____   _____   4. tetany

_____   _____   5. slow heart rate, sluggish physical and mental activity

_____   _____   6. acromegaly in an adult

_____   _____   7. decalcification of bones, making them brittle and prone to fracture

_____   _____   8. high blood glucose; glucose in the urine

_____   _____   9. Cushing's syndrome

_____   _____   10. dwarfed stature and intellectual disabilities (cretinism)

MULTIPLE CHOICE: Carefully read each statement. Choose the word or phrase that correctly completes the meaning and write the corresponding letter in the blank provided.

1. Various skin and intestinal glands belong to the _____.   _____
   a) endocrine group   c) dermis
   b) exocrine group   d) digestive system

2. Glands that depend on blood and lymph to carry their secretions   _____
   belong to the _____ group.
   a) endocrine   c) neuron
   b) exocrine   d) messenger

3. Insulin causes _____.   _____
   a) a decrease in the level of blood glucose
   b) an increase in the production of glucose from glycogen
   c) a decrease in the permeability of cell membranes to glucose
   d) none of the above

4. Endocrine glands secrete chemicals called _____.
   a) lymph
   b) neurotransmitters
   c) hormones
   d) enzymes

5. The gland that has both exocrine and endocrine qualities is the _____.
   a) thyroid
   b) pancreas
   c) adrenal gland
   d) kidney

6. The body's metabolism is regulated by the _____ gland.
   a) thyroid
   b) pituitary
   c) thymus
   d) adrenal

7. The hormone that represses or resolves conditions of inflammation is _____.
   a) estrogen
   b) thyroxin
   c) adrenaline
   d) cortisol

8. The pituitary gland is called the master gland because it _____.
   a) maintains the blood pressure
   b) is situated at the base of the brain
   c) maintains the body's fluid balance
   d) regulates and coordinates the functions of all other glands

9. It is known that the action of the thymus hormone is related to _____.
   a) ovulation
   b) antibody production
   c) carbohydrate metabolism
   d) distribution of hair over the body

10. A deficiency in the hormone from the parathyroid gland will produce _____.
    a) dwarfism
    b) cretinism
    c) decrease of potassium in the blood
    d) imbalance in the calcium level of the body

11. A person having an increase in the production of thyroxin would be most likely to have _____.
    a) an increase in the level of blood sugar
    b) a decrease in blood pressure
    c) an increase in metabolic rate
    d) an increase in physical growth and a decrease in mental ability

12. The two hormones secreted by the ovaries are important in the
   _____.
   a) regulation of the metabolic rate
   b) transmission of sex-linked genetic traits
   c) maintenance of water balance in the body
   d) development of secondary sex characteristics and normal
      menstruation

   _____

13. The endocrine gland known as the master gland is the _____.
   a) thyroid   c) hypothalamus
   b) pineal   d) pituitary

   _____

14. There are four small _____ located on the back of the thyroid
   gland.
   a) adrenal glands   c) parathyroid glands
   b) islets of Langerhans   d) follicles

   _____

15. The anterior pituitary produces ACTH, which in turn stimulates the
   _____.
   a) adrenal glands   c) heart
   b) thyroid gland   d) sex glands

   _____

16. The thyroid gland requires adequate _____ in the blood for the
   synthesis of thyroxin and triiodothyronine.
   a) glucagons   c) Cortisol
   b) iodine   d) glucose

   _____

17. One category of the steroids, called *mineralocorticoids*, _____.
   a) constrict the superficial blood vessels
   b) depress kidney action
   c) regulate fluid and electrolyte balance
   d) relax the smooth muscles of the intestines

   _____

18. The female counterpart to testosterone is _____.
   a) prolactin   c) estrogen
   b) progesterone   d) luteinizing hormone

   _____

19. A person born without a functioning thyroid gland will suffer from
   _____.
   a) giantism   c) diabetes
   b) dwarfism   d) cretinism

   _____

WORD REVIEW: Write down the meaning of each of the following words. The list can be used as a study guide for this chapter!

adrenal glands

_____

_____

_____

ACTH

_____

_____

_____

aldosterone

_____

_____

_____

antidiuretic hormone (ADH)

_____

_____

_____

calcitonin

_____

_____

_____

cortisol

_____

_____

_____

diabetes mellitus

_____

_____

_____

duct glands

_____

_____

_____

endocrine glands

_____

_____

_____

epinephrine

_____

_____

_____

estrogen

_____

_____

_____

exocrine glands

_____

_____

_____

glucagon

_____

_____

_____

glucocorticoids

_____

_____

_____

goiter

_____

_____

_____

gonadotropic hormones

_____

_____

_____

gonads

_____

_____

_____

growth hormone

_____

_____

_____

hormones

_____

_____

_____

hyperactive

_____

_____

_____

hypoactive

_____

_____

_____

insulin

_____

_____

_____

islets of Langerhans

_____

_____

_____

master gland

_____

_____

_____

mineralocorticoids

_____

_____

_____

norepinephrine

_____

_____

_____

ovaries

_____

_____

_____

oxytocin

_____

_____

_____

pancreas

_____

_____

_____

parathormone

_____

_____

_____

parathyroid glands

_____

_____

_____

pituitary gland

_____

_____

_____

prolactin

_____

_____

_____

testes

_____

_____

_____

testosterone

_____

_____

_____

tetany

_____

_____

_____

thyroid gland

_____

_____

_____

TSH

_____

_____

_____

thyroxin

_____

_____

_____

triiodothyronine

_____

_____

_____

SYSTEM 7: REVIEW THE RESPIRATORY SYSTEM

IDENTIFICATION: Identify the structures indicated in Figure 5-23 by writing the letter of the structure next to the appropriate term in the space provided.

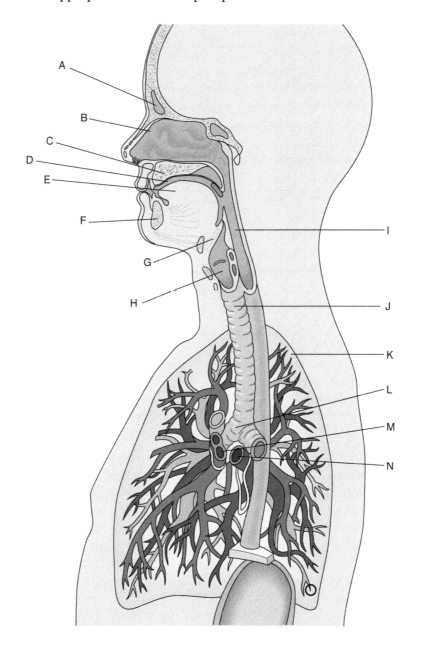

Fig. 5-23 Respiratory organs and structures.

_____ 1. bronchus   _____ 6. lung   _____ 11. sinuses

_____ 2. roof of mouth   _____ 7. nasal passage   _____ 12. pharynx

_____ 3. lower jawbone   _____ 8. oral cavity   _____ 13. pulmonary artery

_____ 4. epiglottis   _____ 9. tongue   _____ 14. trachea

_____ 5. larynx   _____ 10. pulmonary vein

FILL-IN-THE-BLANK: In the space(s) provided, write the word(s) that correctly complete(s) each statement.

1. The exchange of oxygen and carbon dioxide that takes place in the body is called _____.

2. The exchange between the external environment and the blood that takes place in the lungs is termed _____.

3. The gaseous exchange between the blood and the cells of the body is termed _____.

4. The oxidation that occurs within the cell is termed _____.

5. Air enters the nasal cavity through the _____.

6. The function of the nasal cavity is to _____, _____, and _____ the air.

7. The passageway common to the digestive system and the respiratory system that is also referred to as the throat is called the _____.

8. The air passes through the voice box or the _____.

9. In the chest, the windpipe or _____ divides into two _____.

10. The entire system of multibranched air passages is called the _____.

11. The air passages terminate in clusters of air sacs called _____.

12. The act of ventilation is accomplished by _____.

TRUE OR FALSE: If the following statements are true, write *true* in the space provided. If they are false, replace the italicized word with one that makes the statement true.

_____ 1. The blood in the pulmonary arteries has a high concentration of *oxygen*.

_____ 2. Oxygen moves from the lungs to the blood by *diffusion*.

_____ 3. The by-products of *internal respiration* are water, carbon dioxide, and energy.

_____ 4. *Carbon dioxide* is carried by hemoglobin in the red blood cells of the blood.

_____ 5. When the diaphragm contracts, it causes a person to *exhale*.

MULTIPLE CHOICE: Carefully read each statement. Choose the word or phrase that correctly completes the meaning and write the corresponding letter in the blank provided.

1. Exchange of carbon dioxide and oxygen is called _____.
   a) respiration
   b) relaxation
   c) oxidation
   d) ventilation

   _____

2. Internal respiration occurs between the blood and the _____.
   a) cells
   b) air
   c) lymph
   d) lungs

   _____

3. Oxygen is carried from the lungs to body cells by linking (chemically bonding) with _____.
   a) carbaminohemoglobin
   b) hydrogen ions
   c) hemoglobin
   d) carbonic acid

   _____

4. Normal adult respiration occurs this many times per minute.
   a) 10 to 15
   b) 25 to 30
   c) 10 to 20
   d) 40 to 50

   _____

5. When the diaphragm contracts, it _____.
   a) pushes upward against the lungs and causes them to deflate
   b) pulls down, allowing the lungs to expand and fill with air
   c) causes the intercostal muscles to relax and expand the chest wall
   d) pushes downward and inward, causing the lungs to deflate and expel air

   _____

6. The main way in which gas exchange happens through the respiratory membrane is by _____.
   a) infusion
   b) evaporation
   c) diffusion
   d) radiation

   _____

7. A by-product of cellular respiration is _____.
   a) carbon dioxide
   b) heat
   c) water
   d) all of the above

   _____

WORD REVIEW: Write down the meaning of each of the following words. The list can be used as a study guide for this chapter!

alveoli

_____

_____

_____

cellular respiration

_____

_____

_____

diaphragm

_____

_____

_____

exhalation

_____

_____

_____

external respiration

_____

_____

_____

inhalation

_____

_____

_____

internal respiration

_____

_____

_____

larynx

_____

_____

_____

nasal cavity

_____

_____

_____

pharynx

_____

_____

_____

respiration

_____

_____

_____

trachea

_____

_____

_____

SYSTEM 8: REVIEW THE DIGESTIVE SYSTEM

FILL-IN-THE-BLANK: In the space(s) provided, write the word(s) that correctly complete(s) each statement.

1. The process of converting food into substances capable of nourishing cells is

   _____.

2. The process in which the digested nutrients are transferred from the intestines to the blood or lymph vessels to be transported to the cells is _____.

3. The muscular tube that goes from the lips to the anus is the _____ or the

   _____.

4. Organs, such as the pancreas, that aid digestion but are located outside the digestive tract are known as _____ digestive organs.

5. The physical activity of digestion that takes place in the mouth is called

   _____.

6. The chemical digestive activity that takes place in the mouth is from secretions by the

   _____.

7. The physical or mechanical activity in the alimentary canal is from the action of the

   _____.

IDENTIFICATION: Identify the structures indicated in Figure 5-24 by writing the correct terms in the numbered space that corresponds to the number on the figure.

1. _____   7. _____

2. _____   8. _____

3. _____   9. _____

4. _____   10. _____

5. _____   11. _____

6. _____   12. _____

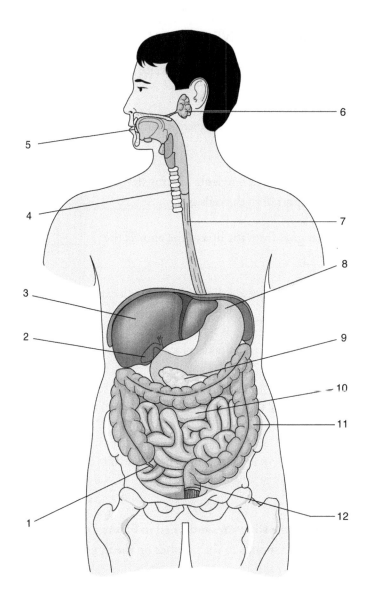

Fig. 5-24 The digestive system.

MATCHING: Match the term with the best description. Write the letter of the appropriate term in the space provided.

A. bolus

B. cardiac sphincter

C. cecum

D. chyme

E. colon

F. duodenum

G. ileocecal valve

H. ileum

I. lacteals

J. mucosa

K. oral cavity

L. peristalsis

M. pyloric sphincter

N. rectum

O. saliva

P. serous layer

Q. submucosa

R. villi

_____ 1. beginning of the large intestine

_____ 2. contains enzymes that begin to break down carbohydrates

_____ 3. a mixture of digestive juices, mucus, and food material

_____ 4. a soft food ball that is swallowed

_____ 5. prevents movement from the large intestine to the small intestine

_____ 6. outer covering of the intestine that is continuous with the peritoneum lining the abdominal cavity

_____ 7. rhythmic, wavelike, muscular motion

_____ 8. opening at the top of the stomach

_____ 9. temporary storage of solid waste

_____ 10. a membrane made up of epithelial cells that carry on secretion and absorption

_____ 11. where food is masticated

_____ 12. plays an important role in determining how long food is held in the stomach

_____ 13. first section of the small intestine

_____ 14. stores, forms, and excretes waste products; regulates the body's water balance

_____ 15. fingerlike projections that increase the surface area of small intestines

_____ 16. organ that receives bile and pancreatic juices

_____ 17. lymph capillaries in the small intestine

_____ 18. serves to nourish the surrounding tissues and carry away the absorbed material

_____ 19. last section of the small intestine

_____ 20. organ responsible for water absorption and feces formation

MULTIPLE CHOICE: Carefully read each statement. Choose the word or phrase that correctly completes the meaning and write the corresponding letter in the blank provided.

1. The alimentary canal includes (not counting any accessory organs) _____.
   a) mouth, teeth, throat, stomach, and large intestines
   b) mouth, throat, pancreas, gallbladder, and large intestines
   c) mouth, pharynx, esophagus, stomach, small and large intestines
   d) mouth, pharynx, pancreas, vermiform appendix, small and large intestines

2. Transfer of nutrients from the intestines to the blood or lymph is called _____.
   a) absorption   c) nutrition
   b) digestion   d) osmosis

3. The small intestine consists of three parts that, beginning at the stomach, appear in the following order.
   a) ileum, duodenum, jejunum
   b) duodenum, jejunum, ileum
   c) jejunum, ileum, duodenum
   d) duodenum, ileum, jejunum

4. The total length of the adult alimentary canal is about _____.
   a) 25 times as long as a person's height
   b) five times as long as a person's height
   c) 50 times as long as a person's height
   d) twice as long as a person's height

5. The wavelike muscular movement that propels material through the alimentary canal is _____.
   a) initiated by swallowing
   b) a reflexive action caused by the presence of material in the canal
   c) called *peristalsis*
   d) all of the above

6. Bile is important in digestion because it _____.
   a) digests simple fats
   b) changes complex sugars to glucose
   c) dissolves meat fibers and makes them easiest to digest
   d) breaks down fat globules so that they can be more easily digested by enzymes

7. The sphincter between the esophagus and the stomach is called the
   _____ sphincter.   _____
   a) pyloric   c) ileocecal
   b) cardiac   d) anal

8. The structure at the junction of the large and small intestines that
   controls the passage of feces is the _____.   _____
   a) jejunum   c) pylorus sphincter
   b) appendix   d) ileocecal valve

9. The structures in the small intestine that are chiefly responsible for
   the absorption of digested food are called _____.   _____
   a) villi   c) caries
   b) rugae   d) ampullae

10. The walls of the digestive system are composed of _____ muscle.   _____
    a) cardiac   c) smooth
    b) skeletal   d) sphincter

11. Food is broken down into its chemical components by the action of
    _____.   _____
    a) enzymes   c) peristalsis
    b) hormones   d) sphincter muscles

12. The organ in which protein digestion begins is the _____.   _____
    a) mouth   c) duodenum
    b) stomach   d) jejunum

13. At each end of the stomach are muscles that relax to form an opening _____
    and contract to close the opening. These muscles are known as
    _____ muscles.
    a) smooth   c) cardiac
    b) skeletal   d) sphincter

14. Enzymes are secreted by the _____.   _____
    a) villi   c) liver and gallbladder
    b) epiglottis   d) linings of the stomach
                                          and intestines

15. The colon functions mainly to _____.
    a) digest fats
    b) secrete enzymes
    c) absorb water from the waste materials of digestion
    d) absorb digested food materials into the circulating fluids

    _____

16. The sigmoid colon empties into the _____.
    a) rectum   c) anal canal
    b) transverse colon   d) descending colon

    _____

17. The parts of the colon in order, from proximal to distal, are _____.
    a) descending, transverse, ascending, sigmoid
    b) ascending, transverse, descending, sigmoid
    c) ascending, descending, transverse, sigmoid
    d) transverse, ascending, descending, sigmoid

    _____

WORD REVIEW: Write down the meaning of each of the following words. The list can be used as a study guide for this chapter!

absorption

_____

_____

_____

accessory digestive organs

_____

_____

_____

alimentary canal

_____

_____

_____

anal canal

_____

_____

_____

ascending colon

_____

_____

_____

bile

_____

_____

_____

bolus

_____

_____

_____

cardiac sphincter

_____

_____

_____

cecum

_____

_____

_____

chyme

_____

_____

_____

colon

_____

_____

_____

common bile duct

_____

_____

_____

descending colon

_____

_____

_____

digestion

_____

_____

_____

duodenum

_____

_____

_____

feces

_____

_____

_____

hydrochloric acid

_____

_____

_____

ileum

_____

_____

_____

ileocecal valve

_____

_____

_____

jejunum

_____

_____

_____

lacteals

_____

_____

_____

oral cavity

_____

_____

_____

pancreatic duct

_____

_____

_____

pancreatic fluid

_____

_____

_____

peristalsis

_____

_____

_____

pyloric sphincter

_____

_____

_____

rectum

_____

_____

_____

saliva

_____

_____

_____

salivary glands

_____

_____

_____

sigmoid colon

_____

_____

_____

small intestine

_____

_____

_____

transverse colon

_____

_____

_____

villi

_____

_____

_____

SYSTEM 9: REVIEW THE URINARY SYSTEM

FILL-IN-THE-BLANK: In the space(s) provided, write the word(s) that correctly complete(s) each statement.

1. The functional unit of the kidney is the _____ .

2. The tubes that carry urine from the kidneys to the bladder are called _____ .

3. A hormone produced in the kidneys that acts to regulate blood pressure is _____ .

TRUE OR FALSE: If the following statements are true, write *true* in the space provided. If they are false, replace the italicized word with one that makes the statement true.

_____ 1. The kidneys normally filter 40 to 50 *gallons* of blood plasma a day.

_____ 2. When a person urinates, *voluntary* muscles in the walls of the bladder contract, forcing the urine out of the body.

IDENTIFICATION: Identify the structures indicated in Figure 5-25 by writing the correct term in the numbered space that corresponds to the number on the figure.

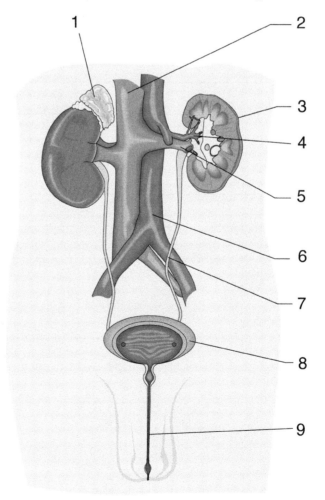

Fig. 5-25 The urinary system.

1. _____   6. _____

2. _____   7. _____

3. _____   8. _____

4. _____   9. _____

5. _____

MULTIPLE CHOICE: Carefully read each statement. Choose the word or phrase that correctly completes the meaning and write the corresponding letter in the blank provided.

1. Urine is produced in and eliminated from the organs of the urinary   _____
   system in the following order.
   a) cortex, urethra, bladder, ureter
   b) kidney, urethra, bladder, ureter
   c) kidney, pelvis, ureter, bladder
   d) kidney, ureter, bladder, urethra

2. The opening between the bladder and the urethra is controlled by a   _____

   _____.
   a) flap-like valve   c) band of cartilage
   b) sphincter muscle   d) fold of membranous
                                             tissue

3. Materials for the production of urine come from the _____.   _____
   a) kidney   c) bloodstream
   b) bladder   d) lymph system

4. The wall of the bladder is composed of _____.   _____
   a) cartilage   c) skeletal muscle
   b) smooth muscle   d) adipose tissue

5. The outer portion of the kidney is the _____.
   a) medulla
   b) Bowman's capsule
   c) loop of Henle
   d) cortex

6. The urge to void usually begins when the normal bladder contains approximately how much urine?
   a) approximately one dram
   b) approximately one quart
   c) about two quarts
   d) approximately one pint

7. The inner portion of the kidney is the _____.
   a) medulla
   b) ureter
   c) renal pelvis
   d) cortex

8. The functional unit of the kidney is the _____.
   a) cell
   b) nephron
   c) glomerulus
   d) loop of Henle

9. Fluid is carried from the kidneys to the bladder by the
   a) renal vein
   b) renal artery
   c) ureters
   d) urethra

10. Of the amount of plasma that is filtered through the kidneys, approximately how much is excreted as urine?
    a) 0.1 percent
    b) 1 percent
    c) 5 percent
    d) 10 percent

WORD REVIEW: Write down the meaning of each of the following words. The list can be used as a study guide for this chapter!

bladder

_____

_____

_____

nephron

_____

_____

_____

renin

_____

_____

_____

ureters

_____

_____

_____

urethra

_____

_____

_____

urinary system

_____

_____

_____

SYSTEM 10: REVIEW THE HUMAN REPRODUCTIVE SYSTEM

FILL-IN-THE-BLANK: In the space(s) provided, write the word(s) that correctly complete(s) each statement.

1. One-celled organisms that do not need a partner to reproduce do so by nonsexual means called _____ reproduction.

2. The term used to describe a reproductive cell that can unite with another reproductive cell to form the cell that develops into a new individual is called a _____.

3. In men, the reproductive cells are called _____.

4. In women, the reproductive cells are called _____.

5. The cell formed by the union of the male and female reproductive cells is called a _____.

6. The gland in the female that produces the reproductive cell is the _____.

7. The gland in the male that produces the reproductive cell is the _____.

SHORT ANSWER: Number the following terms from 1 to 5 in the order that sperm would travel from the time it is produced until it leaves the body.

_____ vas deferens

_____ urethra

_____ epididymis

_____ seminiferous tubules

_____ ejaculatory ducts

MATCHING: Match the term with the best description. Write the letter of the appropriate term in the space provided.

A. Cowper's glands   D. seminal vesicles   F. urethra

B. epididymis   E. testes   G. vas deferens

C. prostate gland

_____ 1. conveys both urine and sperm out of the body

_____ 2. two convoluted, glandular tubes located on each side of the prostate gland

_____ 3. stores the sperm until it becomes fully mature

_____ 4. forms the male hormone testosterone

_____ 5. mucus-producing glands that serve to lubricate the urethra

_____ 6. contains specialized cells that produce the spermatozoa

_____ 7. surrounds the first part of the urethra

_____ 8. two pea-sized glands located beneath the prostate gland

_____ 9. secretes an alkaline fluid that neutralizes the acidic vaginal secretions

_____ 10. secretions contain simple sugars, mucus, and prostaglandin

_____ 11. two small, egg-shaped glands made up of minute convoluted tubules

_____ 12. sperm collects here until it is expelled from the body

_____ 13. located in the scrotum; receives sperm from the testes

FILL-IN-THE-BLANK: In the space(s) provided, write the word(s) that correctly complete(s) each statement.

1. The external part of the female reproductive system that includes the labia majora and the labia minora is termed the _____.

2. The muscular tube or canal that is the lower part of the birth canal is called the _____.

3. The chamber that houses the developing fetus is the _____.

4. The egg-carrying tubes of the female reproductive system are the _____.

5. The glands that produce estrogen and progesterone are the _____.

6. The egg cell capable of being fertilized by a spermatozoon is the _____.

IDENTIFICATION: Identify the structures indicated in Figure 5-26 by writing the letter of the structure next to the appropriate term in the space provided.

_____ 1. bulbourethral gland

_____ 2. urethra

_____ 3. epididymis

_____ 4. erectile tissue

_____ 5. glans penis

_____ 6. prepuce

_____ 7. prostate gland

_____ 8. scrotum

_____ 9. seminal vesicle

_____ 10. testis

_____ 11. urinary bladder

_____ 12. vas deferens

_____ 13. spine

_____ 14. rectum

_____ 15. anal opening

_____ 16. ureter

_____ 17. symphysis pubis

_____ 18. spermatic cord

_____ 19. ejaculatory duct

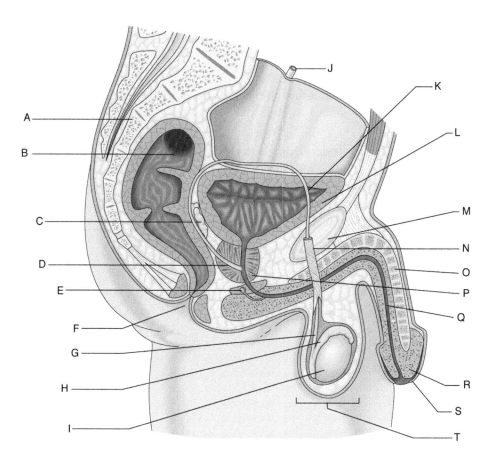

Fig. 5-26 The male reproductive system.

IDENTIFICATION: Identify the structures indicated in Figure 5-27 by writing the letter of the structure next to the appropriate term in the space provided.

_____ 1. anal opening

_____ 2. cervix

_____ 3. fallopian tube

_____ 4. labia minora

_____ 5. labia majora

_____ 6. ovary

_____ 7. spine

_____ 8. rectum

_____ 9. symphysis pubis

_____ 10. urethra

_____ 11. urinary bladder

_____ 12. uterus

_____ 13. vagina

_____ 14. urinary opening

_____ 15. fundus of uterus

_____ 16. ureter

_____ 17. sacral promontory

_____ 18. clitoris

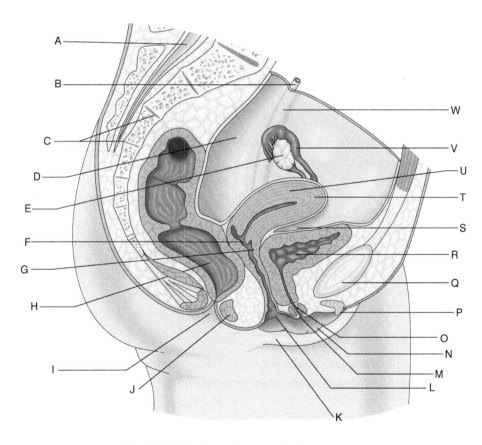

Fig. 5-27 The female reproductive system.

MATCHING: Match the term with the best description. Write the letter of the appropriate term in the space provided.

A. corpus luteum   C. gestation   E. menstruation

B. estrogen   D. menopause   F. ovulation

_____ 1. controls the development of secondary female sexual characteristics

_____ 2. the release of the egg cell from the ovary

_____ 3. ovarian site of estrogen and progesterone production

_____ 4. occurs from the time an ovum is fertilized until childbirth

_____ 5. the cyclic uterine bleeding that normally occurs at approximately 4-week intervals

_____ 6. follicle transformed by luteinizing hormone

_____ 7. the physiologic cessation of the menstrual cycle

MULTIPLE CHOICE: Carefully read each statement. Choose the word or phrase that correctly completes the meaning and write the corresponding letter in the blank provided.

1. Sperm cells are stored primarily in the _____.　　　　_____
   a) epididymis   c) seminal vesicles
   b) vas deferens   d) ejaculatory ducts

2. The hormone responsible for the development and maintenance of　　_____
   male secondary sexual characteristics is _____.
   a) ACTH   c) testosterone
   b) FSH   d) gonadotropin-releasing
                 hormone

3. The upper openings of the uterine cavity join with the _____.　　_____
   a) fimbriae   c) cervical canal
   b) ovaries   d) fallopian tubes

4. Which of the following are canals or tubes through which the sperm　　_____
   pass as they are transported to the outside of the body?
   a) urethra   c) vas deferens
   b) epididymis   d) all of these

5. The number of spermatozoa that penetrate, and thereby fertilize, the
   ovum is _____.
   a) only one   c) at least 3
   b) about 100   d) about 1 million

6. Once the sperm enters the female reproductive tract, it is capable of
   fertilizing the ovum for _____.
   a) a month   c) less than an hour
   b) hours or days   d) more than a week

7. The ejaculatory ducts empty into the _____.
   a) vas deferens   c) urethra
   b) scrotum   d) epididymis

8. The penis is composed of what type of tissue?
   a) fatty   c) erectile
   b) muscular   d) cartilaginous

9. The hormone mainly responsible for the development and
   maintenance of female secondary sexual characteristics is _____.
   a) androgen   c) progesterone
   b) estrogen   d) luteinizing hormone

10. The labia minora _____.
    a) compose the middle portion of the uterus
    b) function chiefly as the female organs of sexual sensation
    c) are two liplike folds situated on either side of external opening of
       the vagina
    d) form a membranous fold that encircles the vaginal orifice

11. The tubular portion of the uterus that extends downward into the
    upper part of the vagina is the _____.
    a) cervix   c) endometrium
    b) perimetrium   d) ostium uteri

12. The physiologic cessation of the menstrual cycle is _____.
    a) menarche   c) a period
    b) menopause   d) virginity

13. Fertilization of an ovum usually takes place in the _____.
    a) uterus
    c) fallopian tubes
    b) cervix
    d) vagina

14. The secretions of the various glandular tissues of the male reproductive system combine to form _____.
    a) semen
    c) mucous
    b) testosterone
    d) sperm

15. The pathway that the sperm travel from the testes out of the body is _____.
    a) urethra, seminiferous tubule, epididymis, vas deferens
    b) seminiferous tubule, epididymis, vas deferens, urethra
    c) epididymis, seminiferous tubule, vas deferens, urethra
    d) vas deferens, epididymis, seminiferous tubule, urethra

16. A cell formed by the unification of a male and female reproductive cell is a _____.
    a) gamete
    c) zygote
    b) fetus
    d) embryo

17. The _____ produces an alkaline fluid that is part of the semen.
    a) Cowper's gland
    c) seminal vesicle
    b) testes
    d) prostate gland

18. Which of the following organs do not contribute to the formation of semen?
    a) seminal vesicles
    c) vas deferens
    b) testes
    d) prostate gland

WORD REVIEW: Write down the meaning of each of the following words. The list can be used as a study guide for this chapter!

AIDS

_____

_____

_____

asexual reproduction

_____

_____

_____

bulbourethral glands

_____

_____

_____

cervix

_____

_____

_____

corpus luteum

_____

_____

_____

ejaculatory ducts

_____

_____

_____

epididymis

_____

_____

_____

estrogen

_____

_____

_____

fallopian tubes

_____

_____

_____

fertilization

_____

_____

_____

fetus

_____

_____

_____

gamete

_____

_____

_____

gestation

_____

_____

_____

gonad

_____

_____

_____

HIV

_____

_____

_____

labia majora

_____

_____

_____

labia minora

_____

_____

_____

luteinizing hormone

_____

_____

_____

menopause

_____

_____

_____

menstrual cycle

_____

_____

_____

menstruation

_____

_____

_____

penis

_____

_____

_____

pregnancy

_____

_____

_____

opportunistic infection

_____

_____

_____

ovary

_____

_____

_____

oviducts

_____

_____

_____

ovulation

_____

_____

_____

ovum

_____

_____

_____

progesterone

_____

_____

_____

prostate gland

_____

_____

_____

scrotum

_____

_____

_____

semen

_____

_____

_____

seminal fluid

_____

_____

_____

seminal vesicles

_____

_____

_____

spermatozoa

_____

_____

_____

testes

_____

_____

_____

testosterone

_____

_____

_____

urethra

_____

_____

_____

uterus

_____

_____

_____

vagina

_____

_____

_____

vas deferens

_____

_____

_____

vulva

_____

_____

_____

zygote

_____

_____

_____

CHAPTER 6

Effects, Benefits, Indications, and Contraindications of Massage

FILL-IN-THE-BLANK: In the space(s) provided, write the word(s) that correctly complete(s) each statement.

1. A massage should not be given when _____ are present.

2. Direct physical effects of the massage techniques on the tissues are considered to be _____ effects.

3. Indirect responses to touch that affect body functions and tissues through the nervous or energy systems are termed _____ effects.

4. Effects of massage on the structures of the body are considered _____ effects.

5. Mental and emotional effects of massage are _____ effects.

6. Any physical, emotional, or mental condition that might cause a particular massage treatment to be unsafe or detrimental to the client's well-being is a _____.

TRUE OR FALSE: If the following statements are true, write *true* in the space provided. If they are false, replace the italicized word with one that makes the statement true.

_____ 1. Friction, percussion, and vibration have a *calming, sedative* effect on the nervous system.

_____ 2. *Active joint movements* increase strength, flexibility, and circulation.

_____ 3. A *conditional* contraindication prohibits administering massage to only a local part of the body, such as local contagious conditions, open wounds, or arthritis, but massaging other areas is fine.

MATCHING: Match the massage techniques listed next with the best description. Write the letter(s) of the appropriate massage technique in the space provided.

A. active joint movements   D. friction   G. passive joint movement

B. compression   E. kneading   H. percussion

C. deep gliding   F. light gliding   I. vibration

_____ 1. prevents and reduces excessive scarring following trauma

_____ 2. rotation of joints through their range of motion with no resistance or assistance by muscular activity on the part of the client

_____ 3. relaxes and lengthens the muscles

_____ 4. prevents and reduces the development of adhesions

_____ 5. contraction of voluntary muscles by the client that are either resisted or assisted by the therapist

_____ 6. helps to firm and strengthen muscles

_____ 7. produces calming sedative effects

_____ 8. enhances lymph flow and reduces certain types of edema

_____ 9. increases the permeability of the capillary beds and produces an increased flow of interstitial fluid

_____ 10. produces hyperemia in the muscle tissue

FILL-IN-THE-BLANK: In the space(s) provided, write the word(s) that correctly complete(s) each statement.

1. Short, invigorating massage stimulates the _____ nervous system.

2. Longer, relaxing massage sedates the _____ nervous system and stimulates the _____ nervous system.

3. Research has shown that an hour-long, rhythmic massage encourages relaxation and reduces the blood levels of _____ and _____ .

4. The positive effects of relaxing massage interrupt the transmission of pain sensations from entering the central nervous system because of what is known as the _____ .

5. The classic signs of inflammation are _____ , _____ , _____ , and _____ .

MATCHING: Match the hypothetical situations with the best treatment choice(s). Write the letter(s) of the appropriate choice(s) in the space provided.

    A. Avoid the affected area.

    B. Consult with the client's physician before proceeding.

    C. Do not perform the massage at this time.

    D. Massage specifically on the affected area.

    E. Proceed with a light noninvasive, soothing massage.

    F. Proceed with the massage as usual.

    G. Refer the client to a doctor.

_____ 1. Miss Harris is 26 years old and has been in to see you on a monthly basis. When she comes in for her regular appointment, she complains of a general achiness, she is slightly flushed, and she has a temperature of 101.5 degrees.

_____ 2. Mrs. Clements asks for you to come to her home to give her a massage. She says she would come to your office except that she has the flu.

_____ 3. Mr. James's wrist is red, swollen, and warm to the touch. He has come in for a general massage and asks you to pay particular attention to his wrist.

_____ 4. Mrs. Annest has come in for a massage. As she is getting on the table, you notice a red, flaky area on the inside of her elbow and another one on the back of her shoulder. When you ask, she says that they are "just some itchy patches she has had for a couple of weeks."

_____ 5. When Mr. Inkles lies face down on the table, you notice a number of inflamed bumps and pimples between his shoulder blades and on his shoulders.

_____ 6. Mr. Johnson, 40 years old, indicates that he is under a doctor's care for a condition that has caused a severe decalcification of the bones.

_____ 7. An 83-year-old woman with noticeably stooped shoulders and somewhat deformed hands wants to start getting massages to help recover from a fractured hip she suffered 3 months earlier.

_____ 8. A 35-year-old mother of three comes in for relief of sore feet and an achy lower back. When giving her a massage, you notice several bulging bluish masses on her legs.

_____ 9. A 28-year-old man comes into the clinic for a massage. He says that he was thrown from a horse 2 days earlier and has a lot of discomfort in his hip and thigh. When he gets on the table, you note a large black and blue area around his hip. He says that he has gone to the doctor and X-rays have determined there were no broken bones.

_____ 10. A 35-year-old woman comes in for a massage. One week earlier she was in a car accident. No bones were broken, but she was shaken up pretty badly. She has large bruises on her upper arm and thigh that are still somewhat discolored.

_____ 11. A woman who is 7 months pregnant comes in and wants a massage because she is "stressed out." You notice that her hands and feet are somewhat swollen. When you press a finger into her ankle, it leaves a slight impression.

_____ 12. Mr. Hill is 54 years old and is under a physician's care for high blood pressure. His physician has recommended massage as part of his treatment. You take his blood pressure when he comes for his massage and it is 170 over 130.

_____ 13. Mrs. Baird is 44 years old and is in the middle of a series of chemotherapy treatments after having a malignant growth removed from her colon. She is seeking massage for relief from stress and "to be good to herself."

_____ 14. A 48-year-old female executive is under a doctor's care for chronic fatigue and mental exhaustion. The doctor has recommended massage as part of her treatment.

MULTIPLE CHOICE: Carefully read each statement. Choose the word or phrase that correctly completes the meaning and write the corresponding letter in the blank provided.

1. Adhesion development and excessive scarring following trauma can be prevented or reduced with   _____
   a) gliding movements
   b) petrissage
   c) friction massage
   d) percussion movements

2. Massage that stimulates the peripheral nerve receptors can affect   _____
   a) pain perception
   b) neurotransmitters in the brain
   c) the autonomic nervous system
   d) all of the above

3. A contraindication of massage is   _____
   a) mild high blood pressure
   b) AIDS
   c) muscle spasm
   d) fever

4. Inflammation of a vein is called   _____
   a) thrombosis
   b) phlebitis
   c) embolism
   d) aneurysm (aneurosa)

5. If a client comes for a massage and has a low-grade fever (100.5° F), the practitioner should   _____
   a) have him drink plenty of water before and after the massage
   b) give them a very light massage
   c) refer him to a doctor
   d) make him an appointment for another time and send them home

6. A piece of a blood clot floating in the blood is called
   a) varicose
   b) phlebitis
   c) embolus
   d) aneurysm (aneurosa)

   _____

7. A mass of blood trapped in tissue or a body cavity as a result of internal bleeding is called
   a) hematoma
   b) phlebitis
   c) contusion
   d) edema

   _____

8. Massage is effective at reducing pain because
   a) it stimulates the concentration of endorphins and enkephalins
   b) it counteracts central sensitization
   c) it initiates the gate control theory
   d) all the above

   _____

9. Massage during pregnancy is
   a) contraindicated
   b) usually beneficial
   c) done only with a doctor's approval
   d) avoided except under special conditions

   _____

10. Body areas where caution should be used to avoid damaging underlying anatomic structures are called
    a) contraindications
    b) endangerment sites
    c) untouchable
    d) landmarks

    _____

11. Stimulation of the parasympathetic nervous system causes
    a) a fight-or-flight response
    b) increased circulation to the internal organs
    c) increased blood flow to the muscles
    d) all of the above

    _____

12. Conditions that require the practitioner to adjust the massage when there are health concerns for which certain massage techniques might cause discomfort or have adverse effects are
    a) conditional contraindications
    b) regional contraindications
    c) absolute contraindications
    d) to be referred to a doctor

    _____

13. Reduced anxiety, an enhanced sense of relaxation, and renewed
    energy are
    a) indications for massage
    b) contraindications for massage
    c) physiologic benefits of massage
    d) psychological benefits of massage

14. Indirect responses to massage techniques that affect body functions
    or tissues are
    a) mechanical effects of massage   c) psychological effects
    b) to be avoided   d) reflex effects

15. The method in which the client's arm is moved through its range of
    motion by the therapist while the client remains relaxed is
    a) passive joint movement
    b) active joint movement
    c) assisted joint movement
    d) contraindicated in muscle injuries

16. Hyperemia is
    a) a contraindication for massage
    b) a condition in which the body produces too much blood
    c) an increase in the amount of blood stored in muscle tissue
    d) an undesirable side effect of improper or excessive massage

17. Massage that increases lymph flow should not be done on persons with
    a) high blood pressure   c) lymphoma
    b) arthritis   d) diabetes

18. If a client has bulging bluish veins on their lower legs, the practitioner
    should
    a) avoid all but the most superficial strokes on those areas
    b) not massage the legs or feet
    c) consult the client's doctor before the massage
    d) proceed with a normal massage and refer the client to a specialist

19. A man in his late twenties comes for a massage. When he is face down
    you notice red bumps and pimples on his upper back and shoulders.
    You proceed by
    a) asking him to shower and especially clean the affected area
    b) continuing with the massage but avoid the area
    c) continuing the massage but using no oil on the affected area
    d) discontinuing the massage

20. A woman well into the second trimester comes for a massage. She complains of fatigue and swelling in her legs and arms. You should _____
    a) position her comfortably with plenty of pillows and perform a gentle full-body massage
    b) give a prenatal massage and send her to a doctor
    c) recommend that she see her doctor before the massage
    d) position her on her side with plenty of support and massage only her back

21. The first and foremost rule of massage is _____
    a) do no harm
    b) refer to a doctor when in doubt
    c) perform a consultation before the massage
    d) get the client's permission before proceeding

WORD REVIEW: Write down the meaning of each of the following words and titles. The list can be used later as a study guide for this chapter!

active joint movement

_____

_____

_____

aneurosa

_____

_____

_____

aneurysm

_____

_____

_____

cancer

_____

_____

_____

central nervous system

_____

_____

_____

contraindication

_____

_____

_____

contusion

_____

_____

_____

dopamine

_____

_____

_____

edema

_____

_____

_____

embolus

_____

_____

_____

endangerment site

_____

_____

_____

epinephrine

_____

_____

_____

gate control theory

_____

_____

_____

hematoma

_____

_____

_____

high blood pressure

_____

_____

_____

homeostasis

_____

_____

_____

hyperemia

_____

_____

_____

inflammation

_____

_____

_____

lymphedema

_____

_____

_____

mechanical effects

_____

_____

_____

nervous system

_____

_____

_____

norepinephrine

_____

_____

_____

osteoporosis

_____

_____

_____

parasympathetic nervous system

_____

_____

_____

passive joint movement

_____

_____

_____

peripheral nervous system

_____

_____

_____

phlebitis

_____

_____

_____

pitting edema

_____

_____

_____

reflex effects

_____

_____

_____

serotonin

_____

_____

_____

sympathetic nervous system

_____

_____

_____

thrombophlebitis

_____

_____

_____

varicose veins

_____

_____

_____

7 Equipment, Products, and Environment

FILL-IN-THE-BLANK: In the space(s) provided, write the word(s) that correctly complete(s) each statement.

1. Professionalism is an _____.

2. As a massage practitioner, list at least four ways to project a professional image.

    a. _____   c. _____

    b. _____   d. _____

3. When operating a massage facility, two standards that must be maintained are _____ and _____.

4. The optimal temperature for a massage room is _____.

5. To ensure an abundant supply of fresh air, a massage room should have good _____.

6. The lighting in a massage room should be _____.

7. A massage practitioner's most important piece of equipment is the _____.

8. Three attributes of a good massage table are that it is _____, _____, and _____.

9. To give the practitioner leverage and to prevent fatigue, the massage table must be _____.

10. A good width for a massage table is _____.

11. A good length for a massage table is _____.

12. One of a massage practitioner's most important supplies is the _____ that they use on their clients.

13. If there is reason to believe that the client is sensitive or allergic to a product or oil, the practitioner can perform a _____.

14. The three main areas of a massage business operation are the _____, the _____, and the _____.

15. To position a client comfortably, the therapist can use a variety of supportive devises called _____.

16. Besides sheets and towels, the practitioner should have _____ on hand to prevent a client from becoming chilled.

MULTIPLE CHOICE: Carefully read each statement. Choose the word or phrase that correctly completes the meaning and write the corresponding letter in the blank provided.

1. The size of a massage room should be at least _____
   a) 5 feet by 6 feet
   b) 10 feet by 12 feet
   c) 5 feet by 9 feet
   d) 15 feet by 20 feet

2. The ideal Fahrenheit temperature for a massage room is _____
   a) 75°
   b) 65°
   c) 80°
   d) 85°

3. Matching massage movements to the tempo of the music is _____
   a) desirable
   b) unprofessional
   c) not desirable
   d) professional

4. The height of a massage table is determined by the _____
   a) height of the client
   b) weight of the client
   c) practitioner's height
   d) size of the room

5. The best covering for a massage table is _____
   a) velvet
   b) suede
   c) vinyl
   d) cotton

6. If oil has an unpleasant odor but is not rancid, add a few drops of _____
   a) lemon juice
   b) essential oil
   c) vinegar
   d) Lysol

7. The primary purpose for a good massage lubricant is
   a) to moisten the practitioner's hands
   b) to moisturize the client's skin
   c) to reduce the friction between the client's skin and the practitioner's hands
   d) to add a pleasant aroma to the massage experience

   _____

8. The time to determine product allergies is
   a) during consultation
   b) at the beginning of massage
   c) at the end of massage
   d) during the second visit

   _____

9. The purpose of linens is
   a) to keep the vinyl from touching the client's skin
   b) to provide warmth to the client
   c) to provide modest covering for the client
   d) all of the above

   _____

CHAPTER

8

Infection Control and Safety Practices

FILL-IN-THE-BLANK: In the space(s) provided, write the word(s) that correctly complete(s) each statement.

1. In personal care services, the three levels of decontamination are _____, _____, and _____.

2. The removal of all living organisms on an object or surface, including bacterial spores, is called _____.

3. Any item that comes in contact with the client must be _____.

4. A massage practitioner's hands can be cleaned by _____ _____.

5. Minute, unicellular microorganisms exhibiting both plant and animal characteristics are called _____.

6. Beneficial and harmless bacteria that perform useful functions are termed _____.

7. Bacteria that cause or produce disease are termed _____.

8. Three general forms of pathogenic bacteria are _____, _____, and _____.

9. The body's natural ability to resist infection is _____.

10. The body's most important defense against invasion of harmful bacteria is the _____.

11. Proteins that are produced in the body in response to contact with an invading bacteria are _____.

12. Submicroscopic parasitic agents that invade living cells and are capable of transmitting disease are called _____.

13. The primary precaution in infection control is thorough _____.

14. An acceptable way to clean linens is to wash them in hot, soapy water and add the correct amount of _____, according to the product label.

SHORT ANSWER: In the spaces provided, write short answers to the following questions.

1. If there is a potential for direct contact with blood, non-intact skin or other bodily fluids, what should the practitioner do?

   _____

2. When should the massage practitioner wash her hands?

   _____

3. List three common disinfectants.

   a. _____

   b. _____

   c. _____

4. List two agents that can be used to disinfect implements.

   a. _____

   b. _____

5. The primary precaution for infection control in the massage practice is

   _____

MATCHING: Match the infection control practice with the given situation. Write the letter or letters of the appropriate procedure in the space provided. Some letters may not be used.

A. boiling in water   E. rinsing with alcohol solution

B. chlorine bleach   F. soap and warm water

C. EPA-registered disinfectant   G. hot water and detergent

D. immersing in quats

_____ 1. to clean a massage table surface

_____ 2. to clean a massage table, face cradle

_____ 3. to clean practitioner's hands before a massage

_____ 4. to clean practitioner's hands after a massage

_____ 5. to disinfect the bathroom sink

_____ 6. to disinfect the bathroom floor

_____ 7. to disinfect the shower stall

_____ 8. to clean linens after use on clients

_____ 9. to disinfect brushes and combs kept for client use

_____ 10. to clean towels used for wraps and hydrotherapy

MULTIPLE CHOICE: Carefully read each statement. Choose the word or phrase that correctly completes the meaning and write the corresponding letter in the blank provided.

1. Every state protects the public health through   _____
   a) commissions   c) sanitation
   b) laws   d) inspections

2. Disease-producing bacteria are termed   _____
   a) nonpathogenic   c) viruses
   b) pathogenic   d) antibodies

3. The mode of decontamination that destroys microorganisms,   _____
   including bacterial spores, is
   a) antiseptics   c) disinfecting
   b) sanitation   d) sterilization

4. The practitioner's hands should be washed before client contact using   _____
   a) disinfectant   c) alcohol
   b) liquid soap   d) detergent

5. One of the body's most important defenses against the invasion of   _____
   harmful bacteria is
   a) healthy skin   c) clean hands
   b) good teeth   d) drinking liquids

6. A sign that the body is working to destroy harmful microorganisms is   _____
   a) infection   c) immunity
   b) fluid retention   d) inflammation

7. Germicides that are formulated for use on the skin are _____   _____
   a) disinfectants   c) antiseptics
   b) sanitary   d) sterilizing

8. To disinfect linens, add _____ to wash water.
   a) chlorine bleach   c) detergent
   b) ammonia   d) Lysol

9. Hands can be cleaned with
   a) quats   c) disinfectant
   b) soap and water   d) bleach

10. Sheets and towels with a rancid odor should be
    a) discarded   c) softened
    b) bleached   d) washed

11. Using proper lifting techniques when moving equipment or clients is
    an example of _____
    a) first aid   c) equipment safety
    b) product liability   d) personal safety

12. When going on an outcall, you should always
    a) bring extra towels   c) wear warm clothes
    b) tell someone your destination   d) drive yourself

13. Which level of infection control is recommended for the hands before
    giving a massage?
    a) disinfecting   c) sterilizing
    b) cleaning   d) none of the above

14. One of the primary ways to prevent the spread of disease is
    a) use a good air-filtering system
    b) use disposable cups
    c) regularly wash hands with soap and water
    d) rinse your hands with alcohol

15. Pathogens enter the body in varied ways that can be called paths of
    a) arrival   c) reproduction
    b) manifestation   d) transmission

16. If you suspect that your linens have been contaminated by a client
    with an infectious condition, you should _____
    a) launder them in hot water and detergent
    b) add bleach to the wash
    c) dry them in a hot dryer
    d) all of the above

17. The practitioner's hands should be washed after working on an HIV-infected person with
    a) a liquid soap
    b) chlorine bleach
    c) a sterilizing agent
    d) all of the above

    _____

18. A class of proteins that serve to protect the body against invading bacteria are called
    a) antigens
    b) antibodies
    c) pathogens
    d) lymphocytes

    _____

19. Organisms that feed, grow, and shelter on another organism without contributing to the survival of that organism are _____.
    a) antibodies
    b) antigens
    c) bacteria
    d) parasites

    _____

WORD REVIEW: Write down the meaning of each of the following words and titles. The list can be used later as a study guide for this chapter!

allergy

_____

_____

_____

antibodies

_____

_____

_____

antigen

_____

_____

_____

antiseptics

_____

_____

_____

bacteria

_____

_____

_____

clean (cleaning)

_____

_____

_____

congenital

_____

_____

_____

decontamination

_____

_____

_____

disease

_____

_____

_____

disinfectant container

_____

_____

_____

disinfectants

_____

_____

_____

disinfection

_____

_____

_____

fomite

_____

_____

_____

fungi

_____

_____

_____

immunity

_____

_____

_____

infection

_____

_____

_____

infection control

_____

_____

_____

infectious agent

_____

_____

_____

mode of transmission

_____

_____

_____

nonpathogenic

_____

_____

_____

pathogenic

_____

_____

_____

pathogen

_____

_____

_____

phenolic disinfectants

_____

_____

_____

quaternary ammonium compounds

_____

_____

_____

safety

_____

_____

_____

safety data sheet (SDS)

_____

_____

_____

scabies

_____

_____

_____

sodium hypochlorite

_____

_____

_____

sterilization

_____

_____

_____

standard precaution

_____

_____

_____

_____

_____

virus

_____

_____

_____

CHAPTER

9

Consultation and Documentation

FILL-IN-THE-BLANK: In the space(s) provided, write the word(s) that correctly complete(s) each statement.

1. A meeting between the prospective client and the practitioner, in which views are discussed and valuable information is exchanged is called a _____.

2. For a consultation to be effective, there must be clear _____ between the client and the practitioner.

3. The two most effective ways for the practitioner to ask questions of the client are _____ and _____ .

SHORT ANSWER: In the spaces provided, write short answers to the following questions.

1. List seven things that the therapist can accomplish during the consultation.

    a. _____

    b. _____

    c. _____

    d. _____

    e. _____

    f. _____

    g. _____

2. When making a first appointment with a prospective client, what are the three questions that can be asked for screening?

    a. _____

    b. _____

    c. _____

3. List four areas that a practitioner may include in a policy statement.

a. _____

b. _____

c. _____

d. _____

4. List three reasons to perform a preliminary assessment.

a. _____

b. _____

c. _____

5. List five topics that should be included in the massage policies and procedures.

a. _____

b. _____

c. _____

d. _____

e. _____

6. List six topics that should be included as business policies.

a. _____

b. _____

c. _____

d. _____

e. _____

f. _____

7. List four topics of disclosure that the therapist must provide to obtain informed consent from the client.

a. _____

b. _____

c. _____

d. _____

_____

FILL-IN-THE-BLANK: In the space(s) provided, write the word(s) that correctly complete(s) each statement.

1. To help to disclose problems and the physiologic basis for the client's complaints, an assessment includes _____ , _____ , and _____ .

2. Information gained from intake and medical history forms, answers to questions, and descriptions the client offers are the basis for the _____ .

3. Noticing how clients hold their bodies, how they move, and how they react to questions or manipulative tests are part of _____ .

4. Various manipulative and verbal tests that help to determine more precisely the tissues or conditions involved are part of the _____ .

5. The outline that a practitioner develops and follows when giving massage treatments is termed a _____ .

SHORT ANSWER: In the spaces provided, write short answers to the following questions.

1. List four sources of information used when formulating a treatment plan.

a. _____

b. _____

c. _____

d. _____

2. List four types of information that are kept in the client files.

a. _____

b. _____

c. _____

d. _____

3. Which four types of information does a practitioner record in a treatment record?

a. _____

b. _____

c. _____

d. _____

4. What are the four sections of a SOAP chart and what does each section contain?

a. _____

_____

b. _____

_____

c. _____

_____

d. _____

_____

5. What can the practitioner do to maintain client confidentiality?

a. _____

b. _____

_____

c. _____

d. _____

_____

e. _____

MULTIPLE CHOICE: Carefully read each statement. Choose the word or phrase that correctly completes the meaning and write the corresponding letter in the blank provided.

1. The process of clarifying the appropriateness of an appointment is called   _____
   a) consultation   c) selecting
   b) screening   d) discrimination

2. Client information can be obtained by
   a) consulting with a doctor   c) client interviews
   b) personal history forms   d) all of the above

      _____

3. A thorough preliminary client assessment includes a
   a) client history   c) client examination
   b) client observation   d) all the above

      _____

4. Noticing how the client holds his body and how he moves is called
   a) body mechanics   c) personology
   b) observation   d) subjective assessment

      _____

5. An outline that the practitioner can follow for giving treatments is called a
   a) treatment plan   c) recipe
   b) client history   d) client file

      _____

6. Work performed on a client is documented in the
   a) treatment plan   c) SOAP notes
   b) client history   d) billing records

      _____

7. Accurate records of a client's treatment help the therapist to
   a) achieve better results
   b) abide by state laws
   c) compare progress with other clients
   d) charge higher fees

      _____

8. All client information should be considered
   a) before calling their physician
   b) research material
   c) when diagnosing their condition
   d) confidential

      _____

9. When should the practitioner obtain informed consent from the client?
   a) at the end of the consultation, after adequate information has been exchanged
   b) when a treatment plan has been agreed on
   c) when there are changes in the course of treatment
   d) all of the above

      _____

10. Downcast eyes, slouching shoulders, a bright smile, and fidgeting hands are all examples of

    a) emotional insecurity
    b) body mechanics
    c) body language
    d) nervousness

    _____

11. Which of the following is not part of an initial consultation?

    a) review outcomes related to desired goals
    b) determine client's expectations and needs
    c) provide information to client about credentials and training
    d) obtain informed consent

    _____

WORD REVIEW: Write down the meaning of each of the following words and titles. The list can be used later as a study guide for this chapter!

active listening

_____

_____

_____

_____

body language

_____

_____

_____

_____

client file

_____

_____

_____

_____

consultation

_____

_____

_____

_____

informed consent

_____

_____

_____

_____

medical/health history

_____

_____

_____

_____

nonverbal communication

_____

_____

_____

_____

policies and procedures

_____

_____

_____

_____

preliminary assessment

_____

_____

_____

_____

rapport

_____

_____

_____

_____

SOAP notes

_____

_____

_____

_____

treatment plan

_____

_____

_____

_____

FILL-IN-THE-BLANK: In the space(s) provided, write the word(s) that correctly complete(s) each statement.

1. Seven factors that control the results of massage strokes are: _____,
_____, _____, _____, _____,
_____, and _____ of the movement.

2. The factor that affects the outcome of a technique or massage is the _____
with which it is given.

3. Four external forces that deform the body's tissues in a positive manner are _____,
_____, _____, and _____ forces.

4. Massage strokes are directed toward the heart to affect the flow of _____ and
_____.

5. The seven common massage methods are _____, _____,
_____, _____, _____, and
_____.

6. Three massage movements classified as a static method are_____ ,
_____, and _____.

7. Four massage movements that are considered to be gliding methods are: _____,
_____, _____, and _____.

8. Four massage movements that are considered to be torsion methods are:
_____, _____, _____, and
_____.

9. Five massage movements that are considered to be shearing methods are: _____,
_____, _____, _____, and _____.

10. Four massage movements that are considered to be oscillating methods are:
_____, _____, _____, and _____.

11. Five massage movements that are considered to be percussive methods are:

_____, _____, _____, _____,

and _____.

IDENTIFICATION: Identify the classification of massage manipulation described in each statement by writing the classification next to the appropriate description in the space provided.

_____ 1. applied in the direction of the venous and lymphatic flow

_____ 2. lifts, squeezes, and presses the tissues

_____ 3. used to distribute any lubricant and to prepare the area for other techniques

_____ 4. manipulation of the articulations of the client

_____ 5. generally the first and last contact the practitioner has with the client

_____ 6. placing of the practitioner's hand or fingers on the client without movement in any direction

_____ 7. rapid striking motion against the surface of the client's body

_____ 8. moving more superficial layers of flesh against the deeper tissues

_____ 9. moving a body part through a range of motion

_____ 10. the stationary contact of the practitioner's hand and the client's body

_____ 11. moving the hand over some portion of the client's body with varying amounts of pressure

_____ 12. used to assist a client to restore mobility or increase flexibility in a joint

_____ 13. raising tissues from their ordinary position and then squeezing, rolling, or pinching with firm pressure

_____ 14. manipulating one layer of tissue over or against another

MATCHING: Match the static touch and gliding methods listed below with the best clinical situation. Write the letter or letters of the appropriate technique(s) in the space provided.

A. superficial touch   C. superficial gliding

B. deep touch   D. deep gliding

_____ 1. Client has moderately high blood pressure.

_____ 2. Client is nervous and irritated.

_____ 3. Client is in pain from severe arthritis.

_____ 4. Client is healthy and has thick, heavy musculature.

_____ 5. Client has trigger points in the neck and shoulders.

_____ 6. Client is critically ill with lymphoma.

_____ 7. Client has stress points in the tendons around the elbow and knee.

_____ 8. Client complains of insomnia.

_____ 9. This is the main technique used in foot reflexology.

_____ 10. This technique is used when applying oil to the body.

_____ 11. Client requests a deep relaxing massage.

_____ 12. This is the main technique used in shiatsu.

_____ 13. Client is generally tired.

_____ 14. Client is visibly nervous and tense.

MATCHING: Match the term in the first column with the best description in the second column. Write the letter of the best description in the space provided.

_____ 1. hacking

_____ 2. skin rolling

_____ 3. aura stroking

_____ 4. active, assistive joint movements

_____ 5. superficial gliding

_____ 6. cross-fiber friction

_____ 7. kneading

_____ 8. deep friction

_____ 9. superficial touch

A. rhythmic pumping action directed into the muscle perpendicular to the body part

B. a stroke with enough pressure to have a mechanical effect

C. applied in a transverse direction across the muscle, tendon, or ligament fibers

D. the natural weight of the practitioner's finger, fingers, or hand held on a given area of the client's body

E. quick, striking manipulations with the ulnar border of the hand

_____ 10. circular friction

_____ 11. tapping

_____ 12. active, resistive joint movements

_____ 13. feather gliding

_____ 14. compression

_____ 15. deep static touch

_____ 16. passive joint movements

_____ 17. deep gliding

_____ 18. vibration

F. help from the practitioner as the client moves a limb

G. moving the skin in a circular pattern over the deeper tissues

H. a continuous shaking or trembling movement transmitted from the practitioner's hand or an electrical appliance

I. very light fingertip pressure with long, flowing strokes

J. moving more superficial layers of flesh against deeper tissues

K. applying pressure with no other movement

L. picking the skin and subcutaneous tissue up between the thumbs and fingers and rolling it

M. moving a flexible, firm hand lightly over an extended area of the body

N. raising the skin and muscular tissues from their ordinary position and squeezing with a firm pressure, usually in a circular direction

O. quick, striking manipulations with the tips of the fingers

P. moving a client's joint while his muscles are relaxed

Q. the practitioner's resistance of a client's movement

R. hands gliding over a body part without touching

TRUE OR FALSE: If the following statements are true, write true in the space provided. If they are false, replace the italicized word with one that makes the statement true.

_____ 1. Massage strokes directed toward from the heart are termed _centripetal._

_____ 2. To have a _sedating_ effect, the rhythm of the massage must be steady and slightly slower than the client's natural rhythm.

_____ 3. A primary indication of tension and dysfunction in soft tissue is _numbness._

_____ 4. The pressure used with a massage technique should start out light, then increase, and, finally, end as *light pressure*.

_____ 5. Deep massage techniques that cause a client to react in pain must be *avoided*.

MULTIPLE CHOICE: Carefully read each statement. Choose the word or phrase that correctly completes the meaning and write the corresponding letter in the blank provided.

1. Most current massage styles are based on   _____
   a) Swedish movements   c) German movements
   b) Swiss movements   d) Chinese movements

2. When a practitioner recognizes the purposes and effects of movements and   _____
   adapts the treatment to the client, the massage practice has become
   a) manipulative   c) therapeutic
   b) scientific   d) resourceful

3. A massage practitioner's main mode of communication   _____
   a) is touch   c) is conversation during the
   b) is during the consultation   treatment
                                 d) takes place after the session

4. A massage movement directed toward from the heart is called   _____
   a) clockwise   c) contraindicated
   b) centripetal   d) centrifugal

5. In massage, placing the hand, finger, or forearm on the client without   _____
   movement is called
   a) static touch   c) intrusive
   b) gliding   d) friction

6. Sliding the hand over some portion of the client's body with varying   _____
   amounts of pressure is called
   a) friction   c) gliding
   b) kneading   d) vibration

7. Rapidly striking the hands against the surface of the client's body is called _____
   a) percussion   c) petrissage
   b) friction   d) joint movement

8. When calming, stimulating, or anesthetizing effects are desired, the
   practitioner should use _____
   a) friction
   b) percussion
   c) deep static touch
   d) vibration

9. A type of gliding wherein the practitioner's hands glide the length of the
   client's entire body or body part without actually touching is called _____
   a) gliding
   b) aura stroking
   c) contraindicated
   d) feather stroking

10. Gliding over small areas such as the face is usually performed with the _____
    a) fingers
    b) palm of hand
    c) heel of hand
    d) elbow

11. Which of the following is not a factor in determining the depth of a deep,
    gliding movement? _____
    a) pressure exerted
    b) part of hand used
    c) weight of client
    d) intention of application

12. Torsion methods or kneading helps to reduce _____
    a) blood pressure
    b) adhesions
    c) stretch marks
    d) arm strain

13. Moving a superficial layer of tissue against a deeper layer of tissue is called _____
    a) cupping
    b) kneading
    c) deep friction
    d) deep pressure

14. A technique that causes an increase in the amount of blood in an area or
    hyperemia is _____
    a) percussion
    b) skin rolling
    c) deep gliding
    d) compression

15. Heat makes the connective tissues around muscles _____
    a) stronger
    b) more pliable
    c) stiffer
    d) longer

16. The preferred technique to reduce fibrosis and the formation of scar tissue
    at the site of a soft tissue injury is _____
    a) deep touch
    b) deep gliding
    c) active joint movements
    d) cross-fiber friction massage

17. A mechanical vibrator that has a back-and-forth movement is called _____
    a) orbital
    b) oscillating
    c) vertical
    d) horizontal

18. A mechanical vibrator that has a circular movement is called _____
    a) oscillating
    b) round
    c) orbital
    d) global

19. When doing passive joint movements, the change in the quality of movement as the limb reaches the extent of its possible range is termed _____
    a) range of movement
    b) stretch
    c) end feel
    d) pathologic barrier

20. _____ is classified as a torsion method in Swedish massage. _____
    a) Fulling
    b) Hacking
    c) Compression
    d) Gliding

21. The technique of lifting and squeezing a part of the body is considered _____
    a) kneading
    b) friction
    c) compression
    d) deep gliding

22. The first technique in developing a therapeutic relationship between a massage therapist and a client is _____
    a) superficial gliding strokes
    b) the consultation
    c) introducing yourself
    d) static touch

23. The intention with which a manipulation is applied influences its _____
    a) pressure
    b) duration
    c) effect
    d) all of the above

24. A rhythmic, perpendicular pumping action to the muscle body describes _____
    a) lymphatic pump
    b) compression
    c) hacking
    d) beating

25. A technique often used to relieve muscle spasms, stress points, and trigger points is _____
    a) light touch
    b) superficial gliding
    c) deep static touch
    d) cross-fiber friction

26. Beating, slapping, and tapping are all examples of which type of massage movement? _____
    a) friction
    b) gliding
    c) percussion
    d) touch

27. The movement of a joint from one extreme of the articulation to the other is _____
    a) range of motion
    b) active joint movement
    c) passive joint movement
    d) stretching

28. The primary indication of tension or dysfunction in muscle or soft tissue is _____
    a) pain
    b) fibrous bands of tissue
    c) trigger points
    d) all of the above

29. _____ is/are done centrifugally with only the fingertips. _____
    a) Tapotement
    b) Superficial touch
    c) Aura strokes
    d) Feather strokes

WORD REVIEW: Write down the meaning of each of the following words and titles. The list can be used later as a study guide for this chapter!

active joint movements

_____

_____

_____

active range of motion

_____

_____

_____

anatomic barrier

_____

_____

_____

aura gliding

_____

_____

_____

beating

_____

_____

_____

chucking

_____

_____

_____

circular friction

_____

_____

_____

compression

_____

_____

_____

cross-fiber friction

_____

_____

_____

cupping

_____

_____

_____

deep gliding

_____

_____

_____

effleurage

_____

_____

_____

end feel

_____

_____

_____

feather strokes

_____

_____

_____

friction or shearing methods

_____

_____

_____

gliding

_____

_____

_____

hacking

_____

_____

_____

jostling

_____

_____

_____

torsion method or kneading

_____

_____

_____

passive joint movements

_____

_____

_____

pathologic barrier

_____

_____

_____

percussion methods

_____

_____

_____

petrissage

_____

_____

_____

physiologic barrier

_____

_____

_____

range of motion

_____

_____

_____

rocking

_____

_____

_____

rolling

_____

_____

_____

shaking

_____

_____

_____

skin rolling

_____

_____

_____

slapping

_____

_____

_____

soft end feel

_____

_____

_____

soft tissue deformation

_____

_____

_____

superficial gliding

_____

_____

_____

tapotement .

_____

_____

_____

tapping

_____

_____

_____

static touch

_____

_____

_____

vibration

_____

_____

_____

wringing

_____

_____

_____

CHAPTER

11 Preparations for the Practitioner

FILL-IN-THE-BLANK: In the space(s) provided, write the word(s) that correctly complete(s) each statement.

1. The study of the interaction of an individual's work environment, tools, and the physical demands of the job is called _____.

2. The practitioner conserves energy and increases power in massage movements by using his _____.

3. The observation of body postures in relation to safe and efficient body movement is called _____.

4. To increase strength and power and at the same time reduce the chance of fatigue and injury, the practitioner must use _____.

5. Regular exercise, good nutrition, hydration, and hygiene along with adequate exercise and regular sleep are part of a _____ practice.

6. The Chinese term for the body's geographic center is the _____.

7. The state of self-assurance, balance, and emotional stability is often referred to as being _____.

8. The concept that the practitioner functions as a conduit or conductor, allowing negative energies to pass out of the client and positive energies to flow in, is known as _____.

9. The most common stances for the practitioner while performing a massage are called _____.

10. The stance in which both feet are placed in line with the edge of the table is called the _____.

11. The most commonly used stance is _____.

12. An exercise that helps the practitioner to reach the full length of a client's body part while shifting weight on the feet and maintaining good posture and balance is called

_____.

13. An exercise in which one imagines turning a large wheel is called _____.

14. An exercise that involves a powerful forward movement followed by a controlled withdrawal is called _____.

SHORT ANSWER: In the spaces provided, write short answers to the following questions.

1. When practicing most massage techniques, where should the practitioner's hands be?

_____

2. In which way does the practitioner apply deeper pressure or more force to a movement?

_____

_____

3. Why is it important to the practitioner not to raise and tighten the shoulders when giving a massage?

_____

4. List seven advantages of using good body mechanics and proper stances when giving massages.

a. _____

_____

b. _____

c. _____

_____

d. _____

e. _____

_____

f. _____

_____

g. _____

MULTIPLE CHOICE: Carefully read each statement. Choose the word or phrase that correctly completes the meaning and write the corresponding letter in the blank provided.

1. The proper application of massage technique uses the practitioner's _____
   a) palms
   b) entire body
   c) shoulders
   d) fingers

2. The most important tools used by a massage practitioner are the _____
   a) hands
   b) vibrators
   c) massage tables
   d) lotions

3. Ergonomics takes into consideration _____. _____
   a) the work space
   b) schedules
   c) tools
   d) all the above

4. The observation of body postures in relation to safe and efficient movement in daily living activities is called _____
   a) physical boundaries
   b) body language
   c) assessment techniques
   d) body mechanics

5. To increase power and conserve energy when giving massages, the practitioner should _____
   a) lift weights
   b) exercise daily
   c) use proper stances
   d) breathe deeply and concentrate

6. Preventing fatigue and conserving strength is achieved through _____
   a) exercise
   b) correct posture
   c) weight lifting
   d) diet

7. Body mechanics does not include _____. _____
   a) aligning the thumb, wrist and arm when applying pressure
   b) the table height
   c) proper stances
   d) breathing

8. The concept that you have a geographic center in your body is called _____
   a) centering
   b) chi
   c) channeling
   d) grounding

9. The concept that you have a connection with the client and can help her to release unwanted tension and stress is called _____
   a) channeling
   b) centering
   c) grounding
   d) counseling

10. Making sure the work environment is functional, and clear of obstacles that may cause injury is
    a) good business
    b) biomechanics
    c) ergonomics
    d) body mechanics

    _____

11. A Chinese term for a geographic and energetic center of the body is the
    a) tai chi
    b) chi
    c) tan tein
    d) Lao Tzu

    _____

12. The practitioner can increase the depth of a manipulation by
    a) leaning into it
    b) squeezing harder
    c) using two hands
    d) breathing into it

    _____

13. Using good body mechanics when practicing massage increases strength and power as it reduces
    a) the length of the massage
    b) the client's heart rate
    c) injury risk
    d) pressure and stress

    _____

14. When performing most massage movements, the practitioner's hands should be
    a) relatively close to the center of the practitioners body
    b) on the same side of the client's body
    c) close together
    d) on the opposite sides of the body part being massaged

    _____

WORD REVIEW: Write down the meaning of each of the following words and titles. The list can be used later as a study guide for this chapter!

archer stance

_____

_____

_____

body mechanics

_____

_____

_____

centering

_____

_____

_____

ergonomics

_____

_____

_____

grounding

_____

_____

_____

horse stance

_____

_____

_____

self-care

_____

_____

_____

tan tein

_____

_____

_____

CHAPTER 12
Procedures for Complete Body Massages

SHORT ANSWER: In the spaces provided, write short answers to the following questions.

1. What is the purpose of explaining your general procedures to clients on their first visit?

   a. _____

   b. _____

2. Ideally, which clothing should a client wear when getting a massage?

   _____

3. How can the practitioner dispel anxiety that the client might have about nudity?

   _____

   _____

4. Why should the practitioner assist the client on and off of the table?

   _____

5. How can the practitioner ensure that the client assumes the correct position on the table?

   _____

6. What is the most suitable position for a woman who is seven months pregnant to receive a massage?

   _____

7. What can be done if a client cannot lie down for a massage?

   _____

FILL-IN-THE-BLANK: In the space(s) provided, write the word(s) that correctly complete(s) each statement.

1. The procedure used to ensure a client's warmth and sense of modesty is called _____.

2. The implement used to support a client who cannot comfortably lie flat on the table is a _____.

3. The process of using linens to keep a client covered while performing a massage is called _____.

SHORT ANSWER: In the spaces provided, write short answers to the following questions.

1. What are three advantages of draping to clients?

   a. _____

   b. _____

   c. _____

2. Which advantage does draping offer the practitioner?

   _____

   _____

3. What is a good temperature for a massage room?

   _____

4. For those times when the massage room is slightly cool, name two things the practitioner can use to ensure the client's warmth.

   a. _____

   b. _____

5. When using proper draping procedures, which part of the client's body is uncovered?

   _____

6. List two types of draping and the linens required for each.

   a. _____

   b. _____

   _____

SHORT ANSWER: In the spaces provided, write short answers to the following questions.

1. To get from the dressing area or hydrotherapy area to the massage table, which covering does the client use to maintain modesty:

   a. when using top cover draping?

   _____

   b. when using full sheet draping?

   _____

2. The client uses a wrap or towel to get from the dressing area to the massage table. Which size should it be?

   _____

   _____

3. Where should the opening on the wrap be located?

   _____

4. List three reasons it is important to maintain contact with the client once it is established.

   a. _____

   _____

   _____

   b. _____

   _____

   _____

   c. _____

   _____

   _____

5. What are two important objectives of a good massage sequence?

   a. _____

   _____

   b. _____

   _____

6. When a therapist is considering a sequence for a full body massage, what are the two primary considerations?

a. _____

b. _____

KEY CHOICES: Write the appropriate key word for each of the massage movements according to the correct sequence in the spaces provided.

gliding   friction movements   kneading
feather strokes   joint movements

1. apply the oil   6. gliding

2. _____   7. _____

3. _____   8. gliding

4. gliding   9. _____

5. _____   10. redrape

SEQUENCING: In the following exercises, arrange the body parts into a massage sequence by numbering the body parts, beginning with (1), in the order in which they would be massaged.

1. Arrange the following body parts into a sequence for a full-body massage. Begin with the right hand and successively number the body parts in the order in which they would be massaged.

_____ back   _____ neck (face up)

_____ face   _____ right arm

_____ left arm   _____ right foot

_____ left foot   _____ right hand

_____ left hand   _____ right leg (back)

_____ left leg (back)   _____ right leg (front)

_____ left leg (front)   _____ torso

2. Arrange the following body parts into a sequence for a massage. Begin with the left foot and successively number the body parts in the order in which they would be massaged.

_____ back   _____ right hand

_____ left arm   _____ right arm

_____ left foot   _____ right foot

_____ left hand   _____ right leg (back)

_____ left leg (back)   _____ right leg (front)

_____ left leg (front)   _____ torso

_____ neck (face up)

3. Arrange the following body parts into a sequence for a massage of the front of the body. Begin with the face and finish the front of the body by massaging the torso. Successively number the body parts in the order in which they would be massaged.

_____ face   _____ right arm

_____ left arm   _____ right foot

_____ left foot   _____ right hand

_____ left hand   _____ right leg

_____ left leg   _____ torso

_____ neck

4. Arrange the following body parts into a sequence for a massage of the front of the body. Begin with the right arm and finish the front of the body by massaging the left foot. Number the body parts in the order in which they would be massaged.

_____ face   _____ right arm

_____ left arm   _____ right foot

_____ left foot   _____ right hand

_____ left hand   _____ right leg

_____ left leg   _____ torso

_____ neck

SHORT ANSWER: In the spaces provided, write short answers to the following questions.

1. In Swedish style massage, an oil or lubricant is used. Describe the three-step procedure for applying the lubricant from its container to the client's body.

a. _____

b. _____

_____

c. _____

_____

2. How is contact with the client maintained when preparing to apply a lubricant?

_____

_____

3. Which preliminary steps should be taken before a client arrives for a massage?

_____

_____

_____

4. How should the client be greeted?

_____

5. When should an information form be filled out?

_____

6. When the client turns over from supine to prone, the therapist holds the top cover and instructs the client to:

_____

SHORT ANSWER: In the spaces provided, write short answers to the following questions.

1. Name three areas of the body where lubricant is usually not needed.

_____

2. Why are gliding strokes repeated between other massage strokes?

_____

3. How many gliding strokes are usually applied between other strokes in a general massage?

_____

4. When applying gliding strokes to the arm, in which direction is pressure applied?

_____

5. When applying long gliding strokes to the leg with both hands, which hand leads?

_____

6. Which special consideration must be given when massaging a woman's torso?

_____

7. When working on the abdomen, what is the general direction of the massage movements?

_____

8. What does the acronym ASIS stand for?

_____

9. When extending the leg during joint movements, why is it important to keep one hand behind the knee?

_____

MULTIPLE CHOICE: Carefully read each statement. Choose the word or phrase that correctly completes the meaning and write the corresponding letter in the blank provided.

1. The most effective way to receive a relaxing Swedish massage is   _____
   a) fully clothed   c) with all clothing removed
   b) partially clothed   d) wearing loose-fitting
                                                  clothing

2. A client's modesty is protected with proper   _____
   a) draping   c) grooming
   b) communication   d) clothing

3. The draping method that covers the table and wraps the client with a   _____
   single linen is called _____ draping
   a) top cover   c) diaper
   b) full sheet   d) wrapping

4. Oil is applied with this stroke.   _____
   a) kneading   c) gliding
   b) tapotement   d) friction

5. The first procedure when massaging a part of the body is
   a) gliding
   b) getting informed consent
   c) applying oil
   d) undraping

6. The pattern or design of the massage that provides for a smooth progression from one stroke to the next is the
   a) treatment plan
   b) procedure
   c) sequence
   d) massage order

7. When developing a massage sequence, which of the following is important to keep in mind?
   a) superficial to deep and back to superficial
   b) adjacent body parts
   c) general to specific and back to general
   d) all of the above

8. A client with osteoporosis should not have a neck massage that includes
   a) kneading
   b) friction
   c) joint movements
   d) gliding

9. Percussion should not be applied to the back area over the
   a) spine
   b) kidneys
   c) lungs
   d) heart

10. When the massage is finished and it is time for the client to get up and off the table, the practitioner should
    a) leave the room and give the client privacy
    b) turn his back to prevent the client's embarrassment
    c) instruct the client to be careful when getting up
    d) assist the client into a sitting position and support the table maintaining contact as the client stands up

11. If a client does not feel comfortable taking off all of his clothes to receive a massage, what should the therapist tell him?
    a) It would be best for the client to remove his clothes.
    b) Draping will be used to keep him modestly covered at all times.
    c) He should wear whatever he feels comfortable with.
    d) all of the above

12. If a client is unable to lie on her back with her legs straight out or head flat on the table, the therapist should _____.
    a) only massage them in the sitting position
    b) refer them to a doctor
    c) support the client's head and knees with bolsters and pillows
    d) give the massage with the client in a side-lying position

_____

13. A reason for placing a support under the chest would be to _____.

    a) take the strain off of the cervical spine

    b) make access to the chest easier for the massage therapist

    c) take the pressure off of the lower back

    d) all of the above

_____

14. To ensure that the client assumes the correct position when he gets on the table, the practitioner should _____.
    a) guide the client as he lies down
    b) maintain contact with the client as he sits on the table
    c) give the client clear instructions before he gets on table
    d) all of the above

_____

15. Low back discomfort when a client is lying on her stomach can often be relieved by _____.
    a) elevating the head
    b) elevating the chest
    c) elevating the abdomen and pelvis
    d) elevating the knees

_____

WORD REVIEW: Write down the meaning of each of the following words. The list can be used as a study guide for this chapter.

bolsters

_____

_____

_____

draping

_____

_____

_____

massage routine

_____

_____

_____

prone position

_____

_____

_____

sequence

_____

_____

_____

shingles

_____

_____

_____

side-lying position

_____

_____

_____

supine position

_____

_____

_____

Cold, Heat, and Hydrotherapies

FILL-IN-THE-BLANK: In the space(s) provided, write the word(s) that correctly complete(s) each statement.

1. The use of heat and cold is a powerful therapeutic agent because the physiologic effects are
   _____.

2. The short application of cold is _____, whereas prolonged application of cold
   _____ metabolic activity.

3. The local application of heat causes the blood vessels to _____ and circulation to
   _____.

4. The application of heat causes the pulse rate to _____ and the white blood cell count
   to _____.

5. A generalized lowering of the body temperature is termed _____.

6. The external application of heat to the body is called _____.

KEY CHOICES: The following is a list of reactions to hydrotherapy. Write the appropriate key letter for each of the following conditions in the spaces provided.

C = Cold application

H = Heat application

_____ 1. hypothermia

_____ 2. vasodilation

_____ 3. reduced circulation

_____ 4. anesthetic effect

_____ 5. increased circulation

_____   6. increased perspiration

_____   7. numbness

_____   8. increased white cell count

_____   9. local muscle relaxation

_____   10. analgesia

_____   11. depressed metabolic activity

_____   12. reduced nerve sensitivity

_____   13. hyperthermia

_____   14. decreased muscle spasticity

_____   15. leukocyte migration into the area

TRUE OR FALSE: If the following statements are true, write *true* in the space provided. If they are false, replace the italicized word with one that makes the statement true.

_____   1. When heat or cold is applied to the body, certain *physiologic* changes occur.

_____   2. A *short* application of cold sedates metabolic activity.

_____   3. The warming effect of the sun is due to *ultraviolet* radiation.

_____   4. The application of *cold* to a fresh soft-tissue injury reduces pain and swelling.

FILL-IN-THE-BLANK: In the space(s) provided, write the word(s) that correctly complete(s) each statement.

1. When a body part is submerged in water, it is called a(n) _____.

2. The application of cold agents for therapeutic purposes is termed _____.

3. The application of water to the body for therapeutic purposes is known as _____.

4. The changes produced by water that is above or below body temperature are considered to be _____ effects.

5. The upper temperature limit for water that is considered safe for an immersion bath is _____ .

6. The normal temperature of the body is _____ or _____.

7. The body's normal skin surface temperature is approximately _____.

8. A bath in which only the hips and pelvis are submerged is called a _____.

9. The acronym for a series of sensations resulting from the therapeutic application of ice is

   _____.

10. The alternating application of heat and cold for therapeutic purposes is called

    _____.

11. When the surface of the body is in direct contact with water, heat is exchanged by the process

    of _____.

SHORT ANSWER: In the spaces provided, write short answers to the following questions.

1. What are the three forms in which water is used for therapeutic purposes?

   a. _____

   b. _____

   c. _____

2. Which properties of water make it a valuable therapeutic agent?

   a. _____

   b. _____

   c. _____

   d. _____

   e. _____

3. The three classifications of therapeutic effects of water on the body are

   a. _____

   b. _____

   c. _____

4. The acronym PRICE stands for

a. _____

b. _____

c. _____

d. _____

e. _____

5. List the four normal reactions to ice therapy in the order in which they occur.

a. _____

b. _____

c. _____

d. _____

6. List four economical methods of applying local cold therapy.

a. _____

b. _____

c. _____

d. _____

7. List three variables that determine the nature and extent of the effects of heat or cold on the body.

a. _____

b. _____

c. _____

8. List the four ways that heat is transferred to the body.

a. _____

b. _____

c. _____

d. _____

9. List five ways of applying moist heat.

a. _____

b. _____

c. _____

d. _____

e. _____

10. Baths can be classified according to the temperature of the water. What is the temperature range for the following baths?

a. cool bath _____ to _____ °Fahrenheit

b. tepid bath _____ to _____ °Fahrenheit

c. warm bath _____ to _____ °Fahrenheit

d. hot bath _____ to _____ °Fahrenheit

e. steam bath _____ to _____ °Fahrenheit

MULTIPLE CHOICE: Carefully read each statement. Choose the word or phrase that correctly completes the meaning and write the corresponding letter in the blank provided.

1. A popular electrical apparatus used to apply dry heat during massage   _____
   is the
   a) heating pad   c) adjustable table
   b) vibrator   d) heat lamp

2. A short application of cold is   _____
   a) anesthetizing   c) contraindicated
   b) chilling   d) stimulating

3. Thermal treatments below 32° F or above 115° F can cause   _____
   a) tissue damage   c) reduced lymph flow
   b) overstimulation   d) burns

4. Prolonged application of cold leads to a physical condition called   _____
   a) freezing   c) hypothermia
   b) hyperthermia   d) freezer burn

5. Heating pads and infrared radiation are types of   _____
   a) moist heat   c) diathermy
   b) dry heat   d) solar gain

6. Hydrotherapy is the therapeutic use of _____
   a) heat
   b) water
   c) cold
   d) massage

7. Saunas and steam baths should be avoided by people with heart conditions or _____
   a) diabetes
   b) swollen glands
   c) arthritis
   d) muscle spasms

8. A local application of cold will _____
   a) cause reddening due to vasoconstriction
   b) increase leukocyte migration to the area
   c) increase the pulse rate
   d) have an analgesic effect

9. Cold applied for therapeutic purposes is called _____
   a) cryptology
   b) cryotherapy
   c) PRICE
   d) hypotherapy

10. Ice is used on some injuries to prevent _____
    a) swelling
    b) bruising
    c) pain
    d) all of the above

11. To increase circulation to an injured area and promote healing, alternate applications of _____
    a) vibration and friction
    b) feathering and kneading
    c) heat and cold
    d) percussion and gliding

12. An economical alternative to commercial ice packs is a plastic bag containing a 2:1 mixture of crushed ice and _____
    a) vinegar
    b) isopropyl alcohol
    c) bleach
    d) antifreeze

13. Water is a valuable therapeutic agent for all of the following reasons EXCEPT _____
    a) it is inexpensive to use
    b) it is readily available
    c) it requires special equipment
    d) it absorbs and conducts heat

14. Water temperatures that are above or below body temperature have this effect:
    a) mechanical
    b) thermal
    c) chemical
    d) psychological
    _____

15. Sprays, whirlpools, and friction are examples of this effect:
    a) mechanical
    b) thermal
    c) chemical
    d) psychosomatic
    _____

16. Cardiac conditions, diabetes, lung disease, and high or low blood pressure are examples of hydrotherapy
    a) contraindications
    b) complications
    c) indications
    d) benefits
    _____

17. The average temperature of the skin's surface is
    a) 96° F
    b) 92° F
    c) 86° F
    d) 98.6° F
    _____

18. Prolonged use of cold applications has this effect:
    a) stimulating
    b) energizing
    c) depressing
    d) dizzying
    _____

19. Expansion of blood vessels following cold application is called a(n)
    a) primary effect
    b) secondary effect
    c) afterthought
    d) contraindication
    _____

20. A bath with a water temperature of 70° F to 80° F is considered
    a) cool
    b) cold
    c) tepid
    d) warm
    _____

21. A bath with a water temperature of 80° F to 92° F is considered
    a) cool
    b) cold
    c) tepid
    d) hot
    _____

22. A cold bath shocks the body's
    a) heart
    b) nervous system
    c) thyroid
    d) kidneys
    _____

WORD REVIEW: Write down the meaning of each of the following words. The list can be used as a study guide for this chapter.

body wrap

_____

_____

_____

conduction

_____

_____

_____

contrast baths

_____

_____

_____

contrast therapy

_____

_____

_____

convection

_____

_____

_____

conversion

_____

_____

_____

cryotherapy

_____

_____

_____

hydrocollator

_____

_____

_____

hydrotherapy

_____

_____

_____

hyperthermia

_____

_____

_____

hypothermia

_____

_____

_____

ice massage

_____

_____

_____

ice packs

_____

_____

immersion baths

_____

_____

_____

moist heat packs

_____

_____

_____

radiation

_____

_____

_____

sitz bath

_____

_____

_____

thermotherapy

_____

_____

_____

vasocoolant spray

_____

_____

_____

CHAPTER 14

Massage in the Spa Setting

SHORT ANSWER: In the spaces provided, write short answers to the following questions.

1. What is the Latin phrase from which the acronym *spa* was derived?

   _____

2. What does the phrase in the previous question translate to mean?

   _____

3. Which elements were included in the *kur* developed by Sebastian Kneipp in the 1800s?

   _____

4. What do Bath in England, Baden Baden in Germany, Montecatini in Italy, and Spa in Belgium have in common?

   _____

5. List the six major types of spas.

   a. _____

   b. _____

   c. _____

   d. _____

   e. _____

   f. _____

FILL-IN-THE-BLANK: In the space(s) provided, write the word(s) that correctly complete(s) each question.

1. In Japan, springs used for communal bathing and personal renewal, including hydrotherapy, massage, and meditation, are called _____.

2. The most popular offering in spas in the United States today is _____.

3. The average age of a spa client is _____ with an average income of over _____ .

4. A spa with overnight accommodations, advanced modalities, and signature services is a _____.

5. The optimal number of massages that a practitioner performs a day in the spa setting is _____.

6. When performing back-to-back massages, the practitioner or spa management should try to schedule a _____-minute break between massages.

7. An ancient Indian system of medicine that uses the application of herbs, oils, creams, massage, and exfoliation to rebalance the body's skin and internal organs is _____.

8. A gentle massage technique that uses light, rhythmic, spiral-like movements to accelerate the movement of lymphatic fluids in the body is _____.

9. A treatment that is given with both guest and therapist submerged in warm (90°–98° F) chest-deep water where the therapist floats, stretches, and massages the guest is _____.

10. The use of essential oils in massage oils, as inhalants, or with other modalities with the goal of affecting mood or improving health and well-being is _____.

SHORT ANSWER: In the spaces provided, write short answers to the following questions.

1. Three reasons that it is difficult for massage practitioners to give high-quality therapeutic massages in a spa setting are

   a. _____

   b. _____

   c. _____

2. What are three things that a practitioner can do to create a sense of timelessness within the very strict time structure imposed in the spa setting?

   a. _____

   b. _____

   c. _____

3. List the main contraindications for heated herbal body wraps.

_____

_____

4. What are three characteristics that body wraps have in common?

a. _____

b. _____

c. _____

5. What are the main benefits of exfoliation?

a. _____

b. _____

c. _____

d. _____

6. Two main customer service skills therapists need in the spa setting are

a. _____

b. _____

7. What are four main teamwork skills required to work successfully in a spa?

a. _____

b. _____

c. _____

d. _____

FILL-IN-THE-BLANK: In the space(s) provided, write the word(s) that correctly complete(s) each question.

1. The term *spa massage* usually refers to a _____ or a _____.

2. A spa treatment that combines paraffin and volcanic mud is _____.

3. It is generally recommended not to use aromatherapy oils full strength or _____, but rather in combination with a _____ such as almond, sesame, grapeseed, or apricot oil.

4. Aromatherapy oils can be dispersed into the air of a room with a _____ .

5. When preparing for an aromatherapy massage, add approximately _____ drops of essential oil to an ounce of massage lubricant.

6. Any spa treatment given with the intention of removing old skin cells is called _____.

7. The upper part of a woman's chest, below the neck is the _____.

8. The principle maneuver for all exfoliation techniques is a _____.

9. A waterproof treatment table with built-in drainage is called a _____.

10. A shower stall with multiple shower heads aimed at the client from all sides and above is a _____.

11. A long, horizontally aligned pipe with multiple heads aimed down to spray a client's body while she reclines on a wet table is a _____.

MULTIPLE CHOICE: Carefully read each statement. Choose the word or phrase that correctly completes the meaning and write the corresponding letter in the blank provided.

1. The spa tradition is thought to have originated with the _____.   _____
   a) Chinese   c) Greeks and Romans
   b) Japanese   d) Persians

2. The first modern spa that opened in the United States in the 1950s and focused on holistic health, fitness, diet, and overall well-being was _____.   _____
   a) the Golden Door   c) White Sulphur Springs
   b) Saratoga Springs   d) Hot Springs, Arkansas

3. The most popular service offered in spas is _____.   _____
   a) body wraps   c) hair care
   b) massage   d) esthetics and skin care

4. Exfoliation _____.   _____
   a) is any body treatment given in a spa facility
   b) is a relaxing, Swedish style massage
   c) combines paraffin wax and fango mud
   d) prepares the skin for better absorption

5. The challenge for many therapists working in spas to give high-quality therapeutic massage sessions consistently is _____.
   a) time constraints
   b) low expectations from clients
   c) inexperienced clients
   d) all of the above

   _____

6. A spa treatment that applies a product to the skin with the intention of removing old skin cells is termed _____.
   a) exfoliation
   b) a skin wrap
   c) a salt glow
   d) a Swedish shampoo

   _____

7. Aromatherapy uses essential oils
   a) applied to the skin
   b) diffused into the air
   c) added to products
   d) all of the above

   _____

8. When mixing an essential oil with a carrier oil, add approximately _____ drops of the essential oil to the carrier oil.
   a) 1 to 2
   b) 5 to 7
   c) 12 to 15
   d) 20 to 30

   _____

9. The primary purpose of an aromatherapy wrap is to _____.
   a) nourish and cleanse
   b) heat and detoxify
   c) relax and improve mood
   d) purge and draw out impurities

   _____

10. The primary purpose of a seaweed wrap is to _____.
    a) nourish and remineralize
    b) heat and detoxify
    c) relax and improve mood
    d) purge and draw out impurities

    _____

11. The primary manipulation used when performing an exfoliation treatment is _____.
    a) long, light strokes toward the heart
    b) small circular movements
    c) vigorous back-and-forth scrubbing movements
    d) short strokes in the direction of blood and lymph flow

    _____

WORD REVIEW: Write down the meaning of each of the following words. The list can be used as a study guide for this chapter.

aromatherapy

_____

_____

_____

ayurveda

_____

_____

_____

bania

_____

_____

_____

balneotherapy

_____

_____

_____

body wrap

_____

_____

_____

carrier oil

_____

_____

_____

décolletage

_____

_____

_____

diffusers

_____

_____

_____

dry room

_____

_____

_____

emulsion

_____

_____

_____

Esalen massage

_____

_____

_____

exfoliant

_____

_____

_____

exfoliation

_____

_____

_____

hammam

_____

_____

_____

herbal wrap

_____

_____

_____

hospitality industry

_____

_____

_____

intake specialists

_____

_____

_____

ISPA

_____

_____

_____

kiva

_____

_____

_____

neat

_____

_____

_____

Onsen

_____

_____

_____

parafango

_____

_____

_____

plastic body wrap

_____

_____

_____

salt glow

_____

_____

_____

sanitas per aqua

_____

_____

_____

seaweed wrap

_____

_____

_____

spa

_____

_____

spa massage

_____

_____

_____

strigil

_____

_____

_____

sweat lodge

_____

_____

_____

Swiss shower

_____

_____

_____

thermae

_____

_____

_____

thermal blanket

_____

_____

_____

Vichy shower

_____

_____

_____

Watsu

_____

_____

_____

wet room

_____

_____

_____

wet table

_____

_____

_____

FILL-IN-THE-BLANK: In the space(s) provided, write the word(s) that correctly complete(s) each statement.

1. _____ therapy has been developed largely by (Dr. John Upledger, D.O.).

2. The layer of the meninges that surrounds the central nervous system and contains the cerebrospinal fluid is the _____ .

3. Craniosacral motion is transmitted throughout the fascia of the body with flexion noted as a gentle _____ rotation and _____ of the body, and extension palpated as an _____ rotation and a very slight _____ of the body.

4. Massage styles that are directed toward the deeper tissue structures of the muscle and fascia are commonly called _____ massage.

5. Rolfing was developed by _____ .

6. Neurophysiologic therapies recognize the link between the _____ system and the _____ system in maintaining proper tone and function.

7. Alterations or disturbances in the neuromuscular relationship often result in _____ and _____ .

8. A hyperirritable spot that is painful when compressed is called a _____ .

9. When a point is compressed and it refers pain to another area of the body, that point is considered an _____ .

10. If a point is hypersensitive when compressed but does not refer pain, it is considered a _____ .

11. The technique used by massage therapists in which direct pressure is applied to the trigger point is known as _____ .

SHORT ANSWER: In the spaces provided, write short answers to the following questions.

1. What are five types of neurophysiologic therapies? One answer is provided.

    a. trigger-point therapy _____

    b. _____

    c. _____

    d. _____

    e. _____

2. What trait differentiates an active versus a latent myofascial trigger point?

    _____

    _____

3. Where are myofascial trigger points found?

    _____

4. How are taut bands of muscle located?

    _____

5. List four common procedures for deactivating trigger points.

    a. _____

    b. _____

    c. _____

    d. _____

6. What are three therapeutic modalities available to the massage therapist to reduce trigger-point activity and restore fascia and muscle to normal functional activity?

    a. _____

    b. _____

    c. _____

7. When pressure point release or ischemic compression are used to release trigger points, what determines how much pressure to apply?

    _____

8. Which method moves the body so that the attachments of the muscle housing the trigger point are closer together?

_____

9. How long is a position release position held?

_____

_____

10. When a trigger point has been released, which action should be taken on the muscle where it was located?

_____

11. What is the preferred method of accomplishing the function mentioned in the previous question's answer?

_____

12. What is the neurologic phenomenon that causes a muscle to maintain a hypertonic state and may be responsible for muscle splinting after trauma is ...

_____

SHORT ANSWER: In the spaces provided, write short answers to the following questions.

1. Who originally developed neuromuscular therapy (NMT) in the 1930s?

_____

2. What are common abnormal signs associated with neuromuscular lesions?

a. _____

b. _____

c. _____

d. _____

e. _____

f. _____

g. _____

h. _____

i. _____

3. Besides trigger points, which other areas does NMT recognize that might be tender when palpated?

_____

4. The main massage manipulations used in NMT are

a. _____

b. _____

c. _____

FILL-IN-THE-BLANK: In the space(s) provided, write the word(s) that correctly complete(s) each statement.

1. A therapeutic procedure that is used to improve the functional mobility of the joints and goes by the acronym MET is _____ .

2. The two basic inhibitory reflexes produced during MET manipulations are _____ and _____ .

3. _____ is given credit for the modern development of MET.

4. All MET practices involve the _____ of the client.

SHORT ANSWER: In the spaces provided, write short answers to the following questions.

1. The three main variations of MET are

a. _____

b. _____

c. _____

2. Which condition responds best to MET?

_____

3. What are the various outcomes from the different applications of MET?

a. _____

b. _____

c. _____

4. MET has many variations in its application, depending on the condition of the target tissue, the condition of the client, and the intended outcome of the treatment. List those variations. Some answers have been provided for you.

a. _____

b. _____

c. _____

d. _____

e. _____

f. _____

g. whether there is passive, active, or no stretch after the contraction _____

h. _____

i. whether to repeat the sequence _____

j. _____

5. Which of the two variations of MET use postisometric relaxation?

_____

6. Which of the two variations of MET use reciprocal inhibition?

_____

SHORT ANSWER: In the spaces provided, write short answers to the following questions.

1. The gentlest of soft tissue manipulations when addressing mobility restrictions from pain and soft tissue dysfunction are _____ .

2. Three bodywork systems that incorporate this technique are

a. _____

b. _____

c. _____

3. How do these three techniques differ?

_____

4. _____ technique was developed by Lawrence Jones, D.C.

5. Describe the main treatment in Strain-Counterstrain technique.

_____

_____

_____

_____

6. Ortho-Bionomy was developed by an English osteopath named _____.

7. The hands-on manipulations used in Ortho-Bionomy are _____ and _____.

8. When practicing position release, which considerations are made while positioning the targeted body part?

_____

_____

_____

_____

9. After the correct position for release is achieved and held for an appropriate time, what is the appropriate way to release the move?

_____

_____

_____

MULTIPLE CHOICE: Carefully read each statement. Choose the word or phrase that correctly completes the meaning and write the corresponding letter in the blank provided.

1. A bodywork technique that attempts to bring the structure of the body _____
   into alignment around a central axis is called _____.
   a) structural integration   c) MET
   b) Trager   d) NMT

2. Realignment of muscular and connective tissue and reshaping the body's _____
   physical posture is called _____.
   a) chiropractic   c) Rolfing
   b) centering   d) Trager

3. Craniosacral therapy was developed by
   a) Dr. William Sutherland
   b) Dr. Bruno Chikly
   c) Dr. John Upledger
   d) Dr. Arthur Pauls

4. A hypersensitive nodule located in a taut band of muscle that radiates pain when compressed is _____.
   a) a latent trigger point
   b) contraindicated for massage
   c) a satellite trigger point
   d) an active trigger point

5. Massage therapists can treat trigger points
   a) by injecting them with procaine or a saline solution
   b) by dry needling with acupuncture needles
   c) with ischemic compression, position release, and MET
   d) all of the above

6. Digital pressure applied directly into the trigger point is called _____.
   a) ischemic compression
   b) probing
   c) stretch and spray
   d) palpating

7. Using neurophysical muscle reflexes to improve the functional mobility of the joints is called _____.
   a) kneading
   b) NMT
   c) MET
   d) stretching

8. The technique based on the theory that as soon as a strong muscle contraction releases, the muscle relaxes is called _____.
   a) contract-relax
   b) antagonist contraction
   c) contract the opposite
   d) fibrosis reduction

9. Positioning and supporting patients in pain-free, comfortable positions is called _____.
   a) transition
   b) MET
   c) strain-counterstrain
   d) massaging

10. Position release techniques _____.
    a) bring the attachments of the affected tissue closer
    b) move away from pain into the body's preferred position
    c) are passive joint movements
    d) all of the above

11. The correct application of the natural laws of life is called _____.
    a) Swedish massage   c) medicine
    b) legality   d) Ortho-Bionomy

12. The procedure that gently moves contracted tissues into the direction
    of contraction while bringing the ends of the hypercontracted muscle
    tissue closer together is called _____.
    a) neuromuscular therapy   c) positional release
    b) tender point   d) reflex

WORD REVIEW: Write down the meaning of each of the following words. The list can be used as a study guide for this chapter!

active trigger point

_____

_____

_____

_____

attachment trigger point

_____

_____

_____

_____

central trigger point

_____

_____

_____

_____

contract-relax technique

_____

_____

_____

_____

craniosacral therapy

_____

_____

_____

_____

deep-tissue massage

_____

_____

_____

_____

flat palpation

_____

_____

_____

_____

ischemic compression

_____

_____

_____

_____

latent trigger point

_____

_____

_____

_____

muscle energy technique (MET)

_____

_____

_____

_____

musculotendinous junction

_____

_____

_____

_____

myofascial trigger point

_____

_____

_____

_____

Myotherapy

_____

_____

_____

_____

Ortho-Bionomy

_____

_____

_____

_____

pain scale

_____

_____

_____

_____

physiopathologic reflex

_____

_____

_____

_____

pincer palpation

_____

_____

_____

_____

position release

_____

_____

_____

_____

postisometric relaxation

_____

_____

_____

_____

preferred position

_____

_____

_____

_____

PRICE

_____

_____

_____

_____

reciprocal inhibition

_____

_____

_____

_____

Rolfing

_____

_____

_____

_____

satellite trigger point

_____

_____

_____

_____

splinting

_____

_____

_____

_____

still point

_____

_____

_____

_____

strain-counterstrain

_____

_____

_____

_____

stretching

_____

_____

_____

_____

trigger point

_____

_____

_____

_____

CHAPTER

16 Lymph Massage

FILL-IN-THE-BLANK: In the space(s) provided, write the word(s) that correctly complete(s) each statement.

1. The Danish practitioner credited with developing manual lymph drainage massage was _____.

2. Thin-walled tubes composed of a single layer of endothelial cells that collect lymph from interstitial fluid in the tissues are called _____.

3. Lymph reenters the blood stream near the junction of the jugular vein and the subclavian vein in an area called the _____.

4. Small bean-shaped masses of lymphatic tissue located along the course of lymph vessels are termed _____.

5. The principal massage manipulations used in lymph are _____.

6. Specialized lymph vessels in the walls of the small intestine called _____carry away a cloudy fluid called _____.

7. Superficial lymph flow is divided into _____ drainage areas called _____.

8. The edges of the drainage areas, in the previous question, where lymph flow separates are termed _____.

SHORT ANSWER: In the spaces provided, write short answers to the following questions.

1. Where does lymph reenter the bloodstream?

   _____

2. What causes lymph to move through the system?

   _____

   _____

   _____

3. The main functions of the lymph nodes are

   a. _____

   _____

   b. _____

   _____

   c. _____

   _____

4. Most of the lymph nodes that drain the flow of superficial lymph are located in which areas of the body?

   a. _____

   b. _____

   c. _____

5. What are the primary lymphoid organs where lymphocytes are produced?

   _____

6. How are lymph massage manipulations applied in terms of pressure, rhythm, and frequency?

   _____

   _____

7. In which direction is lymph massage given?

   _____

8. When lymph massage is done on the leg, where should the manipulations begin?

   _____

MULTIPLE CHOICE: Carefully read each statement. Choose the word or phrase that correctly completes the meaning and write the corresponding letter in the blank provided.

1. Which of the following is NOT a contraindication for lymph massage?
   a) edema from kidney dysfunction
   b) swelling from a sprain
   c) phlebitis
   d) pitting edema
   _____

2. Lymph massage movements
   a) begin and end at the site of local lymph nodes
   b) are circular or slightly elliptical
   c) use a light pressure and slow rhythm
   d) all of the above
   _____

3. There are approximately _____ lymph nodes in the human body.
   a) 40 to 100
   b) 200 to 400
   c) 400 to 700
   d) 2,500 to 5,000
   _____

4. Which of the following carry lymph from the legs?
   a) thoracic duct
   b) right lymphatic duct
   c) Peyer's patches
   d) lacteals
   _____

5. Lymph vessels in the walls of the small intestine that carry away fat are called
   a) fat blockers
   b) lacteals
   c) adipose ducts
   d) lymph capillaries
   _____

6. Inguinal lymph nodes are located in the
   a) cranium
   b) neck
   c) pelvis
   d) abdomen
   _____

WORD REVIEW: Write down the meaning of each of the following words. The list can be used as a study guide for this chapter.

afferent vessels

_____

_____

_____

angulus venosus

_____

_____

_____

chyle

_____

_____

_____

edema

_____

_____

_____

efferent vessels

_____

_____

_____

initial lymph vessels

_____

_____

_____

lacteals

_____

_____

_____

lymph

_____

_____

_____

lymph ducts

_____

_____

_____

lymph massage (lymph drainage massage, lymphatic massage)

_____

_____

_____

lymph nodes

_____

_____

_____

lymph trunks

_____

_____

_____

lymphatic capillaries

_____

_____

_____

lymphotomes

_____

_____

_____

primary lymphedema disease

_____

_____

_____

secondary lymphedema disease

_____

_____

_____

watershed

_____

_____

_____

CHAPTER
17

Therapeutic Procedure

FILL-IN-THE-BLANK: In the space(s) provided, write the word(s) that correctly complete(s) each statement.

1. The four steps of a therapeutic procedure are _____, _____, _____, and _____.

2. Reviewing any information available at the onset of the process takes place during the _____ stage of the therapeutic procedure.

3. Examining the outcome of the session in regard to the effectiveness of the selected procedure for the condition takes place during the _____ stage of the therapeutic procedure.

4. Determining strategies and selecting therapeutic techniques to address specific conditions takes place during the _____ stage of the therapeutic procedure.

5. Recording the client history, examination, and observation takes place during the _____ stage of the therapeutic procedure.

SHORT ANSWER: In the spaces provided, write short answers to the following questions.

1. What are two methods of obtaining a client history?

   _____

2. When does the observation portion of an assessment begin?

   _____

3. What are three things that a therapist can observe while observing a client?

a. _____

b. _____

c. _____

4. During the observation phase of an assessment, what does bilateral symmetry refer to?

_____

5. When does the intake process begin?

_____

6. What is included in the client intake process?

a. _____

b. _____

c. _____

d. _____

e. _____

7. What are four portions of a common assessment protocol used for therapeutic massage?

a. _____

b. _____

c. _____

d. _____

e. _____

f. _____

8. What is the main difference between postural assessment and gait assessment?

_____

_____

FILL-IN-THE-BLANK: In the space(s) provided, write the word(s) that correctly complete(s) each statement.

1. Structural deviations, such as a tilted head, rotated hips, or a raised shoulder, are often the result of _____ .

2. Posture is best observed when a person is standing and is best done from _____ sides.

3. The action of a joint through the entire extent of its movement is called _____ .

4. Three modes used in assessing the quality of this movement are _____ , _____ , and _____ movement.

5. The English osteopath who developed a system of testing joints and soft tissue lesions was _____ .

6. The quality of the sensation that the therapist feels as she passively moves a joint to the full extent of its possible range is termed _____ .

7. According to the doctor's definition, fibrous tissues that have tension placed on them during muscular contractions are called _____ .

8. Tissues that are not contractile, such as bone, ligament, bursa, blood vessels, nerves, nerve coverings, and cartilage, are _____ .

9. The results of testing that the therapist is able to see or feel are called _____ .

10. The results of tests that the client feels, such as pain or discomfort, and the way in which the client reacts to the discomfort are considered to be _____ findings.

11. When assessing _____ movement, the client moves through a particular range of motion totally unassisted.

12. It is termed _____ when the practitioner moves the client's joint through full range of motion while the client remains relaxed.

SHORT ANSWER: In the spaces provided, write short answers to the following questions.

1. When range of motion is assessed, which side should be tested first?

_____

2. In which order should the three modes of testing range of motion be performed?

a. _____

b. _____

c. _____

3. Which tissues are involved during active range of motion?

_____

4. If there is pain during active range of motion, what are the five things that the therapist should note?

a. _____

b. _____

c. _____

d. _____

e. _____

5. If there is a limitation to the movement during active movement, what are two things that the therapist should note?

a. _____

b. _____

FILL-IN-THE-BLANK: In the space(s) provided, write the word(s) that correctly complete(s) each statement.

1. There are three types of end feel that are considered normal. An abrupt, painless limitation to further movement that happens at the normal end of the range of motion, such as knee or elbow extension, is called _____ end feel.

2. It is called _____ end feel, when the limitation is caused by the stretch of fibrous tissue as the joint reaches the extent of its range of motion.

3. A cushioned limitation in which soft tissue prevents further movement, such as knee or elbow flexion, is called _____ end feel.

4. Normal end feel happens at the _____ of a normal range of motion and is _____.

5. Sudden pain during passive movement before the end of normal range of motion was termed _____ by Dr. Cyriax.

6. Abnormal end feel is indicated during passive movement when there is _____ or _____ movement.

7. Passive movement assessment indicates the condition of the _____ tissues.

8. Full, painless passive range of motion indicates that the joint and associated structures are _____.

9. Two indicators of dysfunction are _____ and _____.

10. Resisted or isometric movement is used to assess the condition of the _____ tissues.

11. Indicators of lesions or dysfunction in the contractile tissue are _____ and _____.

12. Another name for resisted or isometric movement assessment is _____.

13. Sensing the difference in tissue quality and integrity through touch is termed _____.

14. A common palpable condition found in muscle that is usually associated with a lesion is a fibrous or _____ band.

15. Examining the outcome of the process in relation to the expected objectives is called _____.

16. The first sense of bind when manipulating healthy soft tissue is represented as the _____ or _____ barrier.

17. The end of comfortable soft tissue movement within the range of motion is represented by the _____ barrier.

18. Movement beyond the _____ barrier would cause tissue disruption or injury.

19. The acronym TART stands for _____, _____, _____, and _____.

20. A condition or illness that has a sudden onset and relatively short duration is considered to be _____.

TRUE OR FALSE: If the following statements are true, write *true* in the space provided. If they are false, replace the italicized word with one that makes the statement true.

_____ 1. Palpation is most effective when used in conjunction with and *before* assessing range of motion.

_____ 2. When *passive* movement and resisted movement both give positive results, contractile tissues are involved.

_____ 3. A *strong* and painful muscle test indicates a lesion in the inert tissue, possibly a torn ligament or fracture.

_____ 4. The more severe the condition, the more severe the *pain*.

_____ 5. *Taut bands* usually contain trigger points.

_____ 6. In the acute phase of soft tissue injury, histamines are released, causing *vasoconstriction* of the capillaries.

_____ 7. In the *acute* stage of soft tissue injury, gentle lengthening and cross-fiber techniques may be used.

SHORT ANSWER: In the spaces provided, write short answers to the following questions.

1. Which information is used in developing session strategies?

_____

_____

2. What takes place during the performance phase of the therapeutic procedure?

_____

_____

3. List the rehabilitative steps for restoring traumatized, injured, or dysfunctional soft tissue to ensure a long-lasting recovery. One step is provided to get you started.

   a. (assessment to determine which tissues are involved and that there are no

   contraindications to treatment)

   b. _____

   _____

   c. _____

   _____

   d. _____

   _____

   e. _____

   _____

4. Which type of muscle tends to shorten, tighten, or develop trigger points and adhesions when under stress?

_____

5. During the performance portion of a therapeutic massage, which techniques are effective to identify abnormal tissues?

_____

6. During the performance portion of a therapeutic massage, which techniques are effective to reduce fascial constrictions?

_____

7. When deep techniques are used, how much pressure is used?

_____

_____

8. List four common myofascial techniques.

a. _____

b. _____

c. _____

d. _____

9. When does evaluation take place during a massage session?

_____

_____

_____

_____

_____

MULTIPLE CHOICE: Carefully read each statement. Choose the word or phrase that correctly completes the meaning and write the corresponding letter in the blank provided.

1. The therapeutic procedure involves all of the following EXCEPT   _____
   a) assessment   c) performance
   b) planning   d) psychological evaluation

2. The purpose of performing a client assessment is   _____
   a) to understand the   c) to rule out
      client's concerns.   contraindications.
   b) to determine what procedures   d) all of the above
      to use.

3. Muscle tissues, tendons, and muscle attachments are called   _____
   a) contractile tissues   c) fascia
   b) inert tissues   d) capsular patterns

4. Bones and ligaments are examples of
   a) contractile tissues
   b) inert tissues
   c) end feel
   d) capsular patterns
   _____

5. When assessing range of motion, first test the client's
   a) painful joints
   b) pain tolerance
   c) strength
   d) good side
   _____

6. Pain and how the client reacts to it is called a/an
   a) subjective finding
   b) objective finding
   c) active movement
   d) contraindication
   _____

7. Limitation of a joint movement because of the stretching of fibrous tissues is called
   a) hard end feel
   b) springy end feel
   c) soft end feel
   d) acute inflammation
   _____

8. The source of pain can be pinpointed through
   a) palpation
   b) hard end feel
   c) inert tissues
   d) range of motion
   _____

9. Determining if goals have been met is called
   a) goal tending
   b) processing
   c) evaluation
   d) assessment
   _____

10. When performing ROM assessment, the order of the tests that provide the most accurate information is
    a) passive movement, active movement, resisted movement
    b) active movement, resisted movement, passive movement
    c) active movement, passive movement, resisted movement
    d) passive movement, active resisted movement, resisted movement
    _____

11. Which of the following takes place during the assessment?
    a) informed consent
    b) client and medical history
    c) deciding which techniques to use
    d) all of the above
    _____

12. Explaining policies and procedures, medical history, palpation examination, and informed consent are all part of the
    a) assessment
    b) treatment plan
    c) evaluation
    d) client intake
    _____

13. Observing a client's ability and willingness to move a body part through a range of motion is _____.
    a) assessing active movement
    b) assessing passive movement
    c) collecting subjective information
    d) collecting objective information

14. When soft tissue is manipulated, the first sense of bind represents the _____.
    a) anatomic barrier
    b) normal range of motion
    c) physiologic barrier
    d) resistive barrier

15. Using the hands and sense of touch to assess the qualities of the tissues is _____.
    a) of little use
    b) termed palpation
    c) represented by the acronym TART
    d) done only with informed consent

16. An injury that begins with an event, causes some tissue disruption, and is fairly recent is considered _____.
    a) a chronic injury
    b) an acute injury
    c) a contraindication for therapeutic massage
    d) a biomechanical deviation

17. When a client is asked to actively flex the shoulder, he cautiously lifts his arm approximately 30 degrees, then stops quickly, winces, and grabs his shoulder. The practitioner should _____.
    a) perform techniques to relieve a spasm in the shoulder
    b) refer the client to a doctor for further evaluation
    c) note the reaction and perform further tests
    d) apologize and continue with a relaxing massage

18. When a client and practitioner have formulated a plan for six sessions,
    a) the plan should be strictly followed for the six sessions and then the results evaluated.
    b) if there is no improvement after three sessions the client is referred to another health practitioner.
    c) slight modifications to the plan should be made according to session evaluations and individual pre-session interviews.
    d) if there are no improvements after two sessions, the strategy should be abandoned.

19. Evaluation is the part of therapeutic procedure that is done
    a) after every session
    b) after several sessions
    c) during the massage
    d) all of the above

20. The four parts of therapeutic procedure include _____.
    a) subjective, objective, assessment, planning
    b) planning, assessment, evaluation, performance
    c) history, assessment, planning, treatment
    d) subjective, objective, history, interview

21. The first part of the assessment involves
    a) performing an interview with the client.
    b) palpation
    c) range of motion tests
    d) all of the above

22. Which of the following should be done during the preliminary interview with the client?
    a) the client fills out intake and medical history forms.
    b) the practitioner asks questions to clarify information on the intake and medical history forms.
    c) the practitioner performs special orthopedic tests on the client.
    d) all of the above

23. Bilateral symmetry and posture are assessed by _____.
    a) orthopedic tests
    b) palpation
    c) observation
    d) body diagrams

24. Resisted range of motion tests are performed by
    a) the client's attempting to move a body part in specific direction while the practitioner holds it in a neutral position, allowing no joint movement.
    b) having the client move through a range of motion while the practitioner provides resistance
    c) having the client lift a weight
    d) the practitioner's moving the client through a range of motion while the client resists

25. When planning session strategies, which of the following should be considered?
    a) the client's request for a relaxing massage
    b) intake and medical forms that indicate back and neck pain
    c) a doctor's report that indicates osteoporosis
    d) all of the above

WORD REVIEW: Write down the meaning of each of the following words. The list can be used as a study guide for this chapter!

active range of motion

_____

_____

_____

_____

acute

_____

_____

_____

_____

anatomic barrier

_____

_____

_____

_____

assessment

_____

_____

_____

_____

asymmetry

_____

_____

_____

_____

bilateral symmetry

_____

_____

_____

_____

capsular pattern

_____

_____

_____

_____

chronic

_____

_____

_____

_____

client intake

_____

_____

_____

_____

contractile tissues

_____

_____

_____

_____

empty end feel

_____
_____
_____
_____

end feel

_____
_____
_____
_____

evaluation

_____
_____
_____
_____

gait

_____
_____
_____
_____

gait assessment

_____
_____
_____
_____

hard end feel

_____

_____

_____

_____

hypertonic muscle

_____

_____

_____

_____

hypotonic muscle

_____

_____

_____

_____

inert tissues

_____

_____

_____

_____

inflammatory response

_____

_____

_____

_____

ischemic compression

_____

_____

_____

_____

layer palpation

_____

_____

_____

_____

medical history

_____

_____

_____

_____

objective findings

_____

_____

_____

_____

observation

_____

_____

_____

_____

pain scale

_____

_____

_____

_____

palpation

_____

_____

_____

_____

passive range of motion

_____

_____

_____

_____

performance

_____

_____

_____

_____

physiologic barrier

_____

_____

_____

_____

planning

_____

_____

_____

_____

posture assessment

_____

_____

_____

_____

postural distortion

_____

_____

_____

_____

range of motion

_____

_____

_____

_____

resisted or isometric movement

_____

_____

_____

_____

resistive barrier

_____

_____

_____

_____

soft end feel

_____

_____

_____

_____

soft tissue barriers

_____

_____

_____

_____

soft tissue intervention

_____

_____

_____

_____

springy end feel

_____

_____

_____

_____

subjective findings

_____

_____

_____

_____

TART

_____

_____

_____

_____

taut band

_____

_____

_____

_____

therapeutic procedure

_____

_____

_____

_____

treatment plan

_____

_____

_____

_____

CHAPTER

18 Athletic/Sports Massage

FILL-IN-THE-BLANK: In the space(s) provided, write the word(s) that correctly complete(s) each statement.

1. The 1972 Olympic gold medalist who was known as "the flying Finn" and who credited daily massage with his success was _____.

2. The application of massage techniques that combine sound anatomic and physiologic knowledge, an understanding of strength training and conditioning, and specific massage skills to enhance athletic performance is termed _____ or _____.

3. The study of body movement is termed _____.

4. In sports physiology, the _____ principle states that to improve either strength or endurance, appropriate stresses must be applied to the system.

5. If the intensity of the athletic training exceeds the body's ability to recuperate, the result probably will be _____.

6. The rhythmic pumping massage manipulation that is applied to the belly of the muscle is called _____.

7. Increasing the amount of blood available in a body area is called _____.

8. If pressure on a tender point causes pain to radiate or refer to another area of the body, that point is considered a _____.

9. The massage technique most often used on trigger points is _____.

10. The amount of pressure that a therapist uses on a trigger point is determined by the _____.

11. _____ is applied by rubbing across the fibers of the tendon, muscle, or ligament at a 90-degree angle to the fibers.

12. The British osteopath who popularized cross-fiber friction is _____.

SHORT ANSWER: In the spaces provided, write short answers to the following questions.

1. Why does athletic massage enable athletes to participate more often in rigorous physical training and conditioning?

_____

2. How does athletic massage reduce the chance of injury?

_____

_____

3. List four negative effects of exercise.

a. _____

b. _____

c. _____

d. _____

4. What are two important effects of compression strokes?

a. _____

b. _____

5. In what direction is cross-fiber friction given?

_____

6. How long is a cross-fiber stroke?

_____

_____

7. What does the acronym PNF stand for?

_____

KEY CHOICES: Choose the massage technique that best fits the description or is most likely to produce the following effects. Write the appropriate key letter for each of the following massage techniques in the space provided.

A. compression

B. deep pressure

C. cross-fiber friction

D. active joint movement

_____ 1. softens adhesions in fibrous tissue

_____ 2. causes increased amounts of blood to remain in the muscle over an extended time

_____ 3. reduces fibrosis

_____ 4. adopted from proprioceptive neuromuscular facilitation

_____ 5. rubbing across the fibers of the tendon, muscle, or ligament

_____ 6. used effectively to treat tender points

_____ 7. a rhythmic pumping action to the belly of the muscle

_____ 8. therapist supports the body part in position while the client contracts his muscles

_____ 9. promotes increased circulation deep in the muscle

_____ 10. popularized by British osteopath Dr. James Cyriax

_____ 11. helps to counteract muscle spasm, improve flexibility, and restore muscle strength

_____ 12. creates hyperemia in the muscle tissue

_____ 13. trigger points and increases function to the referred area

_____ 14. developed by the osteopath, Dr. Fred Mitchell

_____ 15. stretches, broadens, and separates muscle fibers

_____ 16. encourages the formation of strong, pliable scar tissue at the site of healing injuries

_____ 17. based on reciprocal inhibition and postisometric relaxation

KEY CHOICES: Choose the athletic massage application that best fits the description. Write the key letter of the application next to the description in the space provided.

A = Post-event massage

B = Pre-event massage

C = Rehabilitation massage

D = Restorative training massage

_____ 1. focuses on the restoration of tissue function following injury

_____ 2. given within the first hour or two after participating in an event

_____ 3. breaks down transverse adhesions that might have resulted from previous injuries

_____ 4. warms and loosens the muscles, causing hyperemia in specific muscle areas

_____ 5. can locate and relieve areas of stress that carry a high risk of injury

_____ 6. stimulates circulation and at the same time calms the nervous system

_____ 7. reduces fibrosis caused by muscle injury

_____ 8. given 15 minutes to 2 hours before an event

_____ 9. is considered a regular and valuable part of the athlete's training schedule

_____ 10. enables the athlete to reach his peak performance earlier in the event and maintain that performance longer

_____ 11. allows the athlete to train at a higher level of intensity, more consistently, with less chance of injury

_____ 12. shortens the time that it takes for an injury to heal

_____ 13. makes more intense and frequent workouts possible, thereby improving overall performance

_____ 14. is fast paced and invigorating

_____ 15. accelerates healing so that the athlete's "down time" is cut to a minimum

_____ 16. helps to form strong, pliable scar tissue

_____ 17. given after the athlete has had a chance to cool down from the exertion of the competition or exercise

TRUE OR FALSE: If the following statements are true, write *true* in the space provided. If they are false, replace the italicized word with one that makes the statement true.

_____ 1. Pre-event massage increases flexibility and circulation and *replaces* the warm-up before an event.

_____ 2. During *pre-event massage*, adhesions can be eliminated to reduce the chance of injury.

_____ 3. Post-event massage is given after competition and helps an athlete *quiet the nervous system and reduce muscle tension.*

_____ 4. *Restorative massage* can help an athlete recover from an injury with less chance of reinjury.

_____ 5. *Restorative massage* include techniques used in pre-event or post-event massage.

_____ 6. A *strain* involves the stretching or tearing of a ligament.

_____ 7. A *grade I* strain is the most severe.

_____ 8. As a muscle fiber contracts, the sarcolemma and the *endomysium* move as a unit.

SHORT ANSWER: In the spaces provided, write short answers to the following questions.

1. What is the first step when giving a post-event massage?

_____

2. After a long race, what are some conditions that the therapist should watch for?

_____

3. Which action should the therapist take if strains, sprains, abrasions, or contusions are apparent?

_____

4. When interviewing an athlete for determining a training massage program, what are five important questions to ask?

a. _____

b. _____

c. _____

d. _____

e. _____

FILL-IN-THE-BLANK: In the space(s) provided, write the word(s) that correctly complete(s) each statement.

1. Athletic injuries that have a sudden and definite onset and are usually of relatively short duration are considered to be _____ injuries.

2. A muscle strain in which there is severe tearing and complete loss of function is called a grade _____ strain.

3. The therapist's indicator of how intensely to work on an injury site is _____.

4. Athletic injuries that have a gradual onset, tend to last for a long time, or recur often are considered _____ injuries.

SHORT ANSWER: In the spaces provided, write short answers to the following questions.

1. Give six examples of acute athletic injuries.

   a. _____

   b. _____

   c. _____

   d. _____

   e. _____

   f. _____

2. What effect does PRICE have on soft-tissue injuries?

   _____

3. When can massage be started on injured tissue?

   _____

4. List two positive effects of the swelling that results from tissue damage.

   a. _____

   b. _____

5. List six therapeutic modalities used in rehabilitation sport massage.

a. _____

b. _____

c. _____

d. _____

e. _____

6. List three negative effects of the swelling that results from tissue damage.

a. _____

b. _____

c. _____

KEY CHOICES: Identify the following conditions as either chronic or acute. Write the appropriate key letter in the space provided.

C = Chronic

A = Acute

_____   1. dislocated shoulder

_____   2. iliotibial band syndrome

_____   3. shin splints

_____   4. wrist fracture

_____   5. overuse syndrome

_____   6. torn ligament

_____   7. sprained ankle

_____   8. tennis elbow

_____   9. bruised hip

_____   10. tendonitis

FILL-IN-THE-BLANK: In the space(s) provided, write the word(s) that correctly complete(s) each statement.

1. The tensile strength of connective tissue is provided by _____.

2. The layer of connective tissue that closely covers an individual muscle is the _____.

3. Connective tissue extends beyond the end of the muscle to become _____.

4. The perimysium extends inward from the epimysium and separates the muscle into bundles of muscle fibers or _____.

5. Each muscle fiber is covered by a delicate connective tissue covering called the _____.

6. Soft-tissue injuries result in the tearing of _____ in the connective tissue.

7. Collagen fibers are produced by _____

8. Collagen formation that reconnects the injured tissue forms _____.

9. Collagen fibers that connect to structures other than the injured tissue form _____ that restrict mobility.

10. Proper _____ reduces the degree of secondary trauma following soft-tissue injury.

MULTIPLE CHOICE: Carefully read each statement. Choose the word or phrase that correctly completes the meaning and write the corresponding letter in the blank provided.

1. Kinesiology is the study of   _____
   a) muscles   c) body movement
   b) cells   d) muscle strength

2. Blood remaining in muscle for an extended period is called   _____
   a) hyperemia   c) hyperthermia
   b) hypertension   d) ischemia

3. Compression strokes in athletic massage use the   _____
   a) knuckles   c) fingertips
   b) forearm   d) palm

4. An active trigger point causes pain to _____ when palpated.   _____
   a) radiate   c) dissipate
   b) evaporate   d) increase

5. Shaking and jostling are performed on muscles that are _____.
   a) large
   b) small
   c) injured
   d) relaxed

6. The therapist-assisted active and resistive patterned movements used in the rehabilitation of disabilities are commonly known as _____.
   a) MET
   b) PNF
   c) ROM
   d) PHD

7. MET helps to counteract _____.
   a) soft-tissue injury
   b) headache
   c) sprains
   d) muscle spasm

8. Pre-event massage should be given this far in advance of an event.
   a) 30 minutes
   b) 2 days
   c) 3 hours
   d) 6 hours

9. The most beneficial form of massage for athletes is _____ massage.
   a) pre-event
   b) post-event
   c) restorative
   d) rehabilitative

10. A sprain with mild pain and minimal loss of function is classified as _____.
    a) Grade I
    b) Grade II
    c) Grade III
    d) Grade IV

11. A sprain with some tearing of fibrous tissue is classified as _____.
    a) Grade I
    b) Grade II
    c) Grade III
    d) Grade IV

12. Injuries that have a gradual onset or recur often are called _____.
    a) sprains
    b) occupational
    c) acute
    d) chronic

13. An injury in or between muscle fibers is called _____.
    a) macrotrauma
    b) microtrauma
    c) chronic
    d) acute

WORD REVIEW: Write down the meaning of each of the following words. The list can be used as a study guide for this chapter!

acute soft-tissue injuries

_____

_____

_____

athletic massage

_____

_____

_____

chronic soft-tissue injuries

_____

_____

_____

compression strokes

_____

_____

_____

cross-fiber massage

_____

_____

_____

endomysium

_____

_____

_____

endurance

_____

_____

_____

epimysium

_____

_____

_____

fascicle

_____

_____

_____

hyperemia

_____

_____

_____

inflammatory response

_____

_____

_____

intra-event massage

_____

_____

_____

overload

_____

_____

_____

perimysium

_____

_____

_____

PRICE

_____

_____

_____

pre-event massage

_____

_____

_____

proprioceptive neuromuscular facilitation

_____

_____

_____

rehabilitative massage

_____

_____

_____

restorative massage

_____

_____

_____

sports massage

_____

_____

_____

tender points

_____

_____

_____

transverse friction massage

_____

_____

_____

CHAPTER

19 Massage for Special Populations

FILL-IN-THE-BLANK: In the space(s) provided, write the word(s) that correctly complete(s) each statement.

1. Massage practitioners can sharpen their skills and stay current with new developments in the massage field through _____.

2. Massage given to a pregnant woman is commonly called _____.

3. The main goal of prenatal massage is _____.

4. During pregnancy, a woman's body experiences both _____ and _____ changes.

5. Any deep massage directly on the abdomen during pregnancy is _____.

6. During pregnancy, emotional mood swings and softening of connective tissues are caused by _____.

7. Excessive weight gain; high blood pressure; swelling in the hands, legs, and face; and protein in the urine during pregnancy are signs of _____.

SHORT ANSWER: In the spaces provided, write short answers to the following questions.

1. What are two considerations when positioning a pregnant woman for massage?

   a. _____

   b. _____

2. Why is the supine position not recommended during the later stages of pregnancy?

   _____

3. List the major contraindications for prenatal massage.

a. _____

b. _____

c. _____

d. _____

e. _____

f. _____

4. List eight risk factors that increase the possibility of miscarriage during the first trimester of pregnancy.

a. _____

_____

b. _____

_____

c. _____

_____

d. _____

_____

e. _____

_____

f. _____

_____

g. _____

_____

h. _____

_____

MATCHING: Match the term with the best description. Write the letter or letters of the best description in the space provided.

A. first trimester   C. third trimester

B. second trimester   D. fourth trimester

_____ 1. Avoid all abdominal massage.

_____ 2. The baby doubles in length to about 20 inches.

_____ 3. The abdomen begins to protrude.

_____ 4. Massage helps to firm slack muscles and regain normal weight.

_____ 5. Weeks 14 to 26 of the pregnancy

_____ 6. Supine and prone positions are suitable as long as the client is comfortable.

_____ 7. The baby's head drops into the pelvis.

_____ 8. Use the semi-reclining or side-lying position for comfort and safety.

_____ 9. Provide massage only after the mother-to-be has received permission from her midwife or physician.

_____ 10. The mother will begin to feel the baby move.

_____ 11. The mother's body starts to produce the hormone relaxin.

_____ 12. Apply only light abdominal massage.

FILL-IN-THE-BLANK: In the space(s) provided, write the word(s) that correctly complete(s) each statement.

1. The person best suited to administer infant massage is the _____.

2. Three benefits of infant massage for the infant are _____, _____, and _____.

3. A full-body well baby infant massage usually lasts about _____ minutes or _____ _____.

4. The length of a massage for a young child depends on _____.

5. A spinal cord injury in the cervical spine usually results in a condition called _____.

6. A spinal cord injury to the thoracic or lumbar spine usually results in a condition called _____.

SHORT ANSWER: In the spaces provided, write short answers to the following questions.

1. What are three considerations when providing massage services to someone who is blind ?

    a. _____

    b. _____

    c. _____

2. When massage for children under the age of 18 is to be done, name two things that the parent or guardian should do.

    a. _____

    b. _____

3. List three benefits for massaging elderly clients.

    a. _____

    b. _____

    c. _____

4. What are four considerations for providing massage for someone with auditory impairment?

    a. _____

    b. _____

    c. _____

    d. _____

5. When providing massage to someone with paralysis, which considerations are made when massaging the paralyzed areas?

    a. _____

    _____

b. _____

_____

c. _____

_____

FILL-IN-THE-BLANK: In the space(s) provided, write the word(s) that correctly complete(s) each statement.

1. _____, or proliferation of cancer cells, is the manner in which cancer spreads.

2. Cancers that are most lethal are those that _____.

3. The four ways that cancer spreads are _____,

_____ , _____ , and

_____ .

4. The kind of tissue that cancer originally develops in determines the _____ of cancer.

5. Cancer that has spread into regional lymph nodes and/or other tissues in the local area of the primary tumor is classified as stage _____ cancer.

6. Three common medical treatments for cancer are _____ , _____ , and

_____ .

7. Leg massage on a postsurgical patient is a contraindication because of an increased chance of

_____ .

8. Surgical removal of regional lymph nodes can result in swelling, a condition called

_____ .

9. The use of orally or intravenously administered drugs or chemicals to treat cancer is termed

_____ .

10. For a person receiving the previously named treatment, the best time to receive massage is either _____ the treatment or after the adverse side effects have subsided.

MULTIPLE CHOICE: Carefully read each statement. Choose the word or phrase that correctly completes the meaning and write the corresponding letter in the blank provided.

1. When a woman is pregnant, ligaments and other connective tissue tend to soften because of _____. _____
   a) estrogen
   b) relaxin
   c) progesterone
   d) stress

2. During the second and third trimester, the preferred position for a pregnant woman to receive a massage is the _____ position. _____
   a) prone
   b) supine
   c) seated
   d) side-lying

3. If an expectant mother is experiencing headaches, edema, and high blood pressure, she should _____. _____
   a) see her doctor without delay
   b) get a massage
   c) go to bed and rest
   d) drink more water and exercise

4. Signs of a DVT are _____. _____
   a) pain around the area
   b) redness and tenderness
   c) swelling distal to the area
   d) all of the above

5. During which portion of a pregnancy is the expectant mother more likely to experience nausea and sensitivity to some smells and tastes? _____
   a) the first trimester
   b) the second trimester
   c) the third trimester
   d) the entire pregnancy

6. What is the main focus of prenatal massage in the third trimester? _____
   a) pain relief
   b) relaxation
   c) preparation for delivery
   d) stimulate uterine activity

7. The first official director of the International Infant Massage Instructor Association was _____. _____
   a) Vimala Schneider McClure
   b) Frederick Leboyer
   c) Diana Moore
   d) Tiffany Fields

8. The person best suited to perform infant massage on a baby is _____. _____
   a) the primary caregiver
   b) a licensed massage therapist
   c) the infant massage instructor
   d) the baby's physician

9. What is the preferable location to perform infant massage?
   a) In a warm bathtub
   b) At the doctor's office
   c) On a massage table
   d) On a blanket on the floor

   _____

10. The length of a typical infant massage is about _____ minutes.
    a) 5
    b) 20
    c) 30
    d) 60

    _____

11. An important consideration when providing massage to children or adolescents is _____.
    a) their attention span
    b) having an adult in the massage room
    c) their body image
    d) all the above

    _____

12. When a client has a disability, how can the therapist determine which special needs the client has?
    a) Ask the client
    b) Ask the client's caregiver
    c) Ask the client's physician
    d) Consult the Internet

    _____

13. A complete spinal cord injury to the upper thoracic spine results in _____.
    a) paraplegia
    b) quadriplegia
    c) tetraplegia
    d) hemiplegia

    _____

14. Which of the following techniques is not appropriate when providing massage for someone who is critically ill?
    a) superficial gliding
    b) MET
    c) Reiki
    d) light touch

    _____

15. The purpose of massage for the critically ill client is to bring _____.
    a) pleasure
    b) relaxation
    c) comfort
    d) all of the above

    _____

16. Massage for the critically ill client is a specialty massage _____.
    a) in which contraindications do not exist
    b) in which, depending on conditions, special precautions are taken
    c) done only in hospitals and nursing homes
    d) designed to enable a person to regain his health

    _____

17. The manner in which cancer spreads is _____.
    a) through airborne particles
    b) metastasis
    c) by human contact
    d) all the above

    _____

18. Cancer that is well developed and has spread to several organs in the body is termed _____.
    a) recurrent
    b) stage I cancer
    c) stage III cancer
    d) stage IV cancer

    _____

19. Cancer can spread within a person's body _____.
    a) through the bloodstream
    b) by directly invading neighboring tissues
    c) through the lymph system
    d) all of the above

    _____

20. Cancer is a disease that is often spread through the _____.
    a) genes
    b) lymphatic system
    c) air
    d) digestive system

    _____

WORD REVIEW: Write down the meaning of each of the following words. The list can be used as a study guide for this unit.

bonding

_____

_____

_____

carcinoma

_____

_____

_____

contralateral

_____

_____

_____

disability

_____

_____

_____

impairment

_____

_____

_____

hemiplegia

_____

_____

_____

leukemia

_____

_____

_____

lymphoma

_____

_____

_____

metastasis

_____

_____

_____

myeloma

_____

_____

preeclampsia

_____

_____

_____

prenatal massage

_____

_____

_____

primary caregiver

_____

_____

_____

quadriplegia

_____

_____

_____

sarcoma

_____

_____

_____

skinship

_____

_____

_____

FILL-IN-THE-BLANK: In the space(s) provided, write the word(s) that correctly complete(s) each question.

1. The use of massage in the medical field in the United States became nearly nonexistent in the _____ .

2. In the 1960s and 1970s, massage began to reemerge as a part of the _____ _____ .

3. Health-enhancing practices that were outside of conventional allopathic medical practices became known as _____ medicine.

4. CAM is an acronym that stands for _____ and encompasses many healing practices, philosophies, and therapies that conventional Western medicine does not include.

5. Therapies are termed as _____ when used in addition to conventional treatments and as _____ when used instead of conventional treatment.

6. _____ combines CAM with allopathic medicine.

7. The most popular and requested CAM modality at most integrative medicine clinics is _____ .

8. Medically prescribed massage performed with the intention of improving pathologies diagnosed by a physician is termed _____ .

9. A document that is signed by the client and that is required to share confidential information with insurance companies, physicians, or attorneys is a _____ .

10. A standard form recognized by most insurance companies used to submit claims is the _____ form.

11. _____ were developed by the American Medical Association to categorize and quantify medical services accurately.

SHORT ANSWER: In the spaces provided, write short answers to the following questions

1. What is contained in massage documentation in an integrative setting?

   a. _____

   b. _____

   c. _____

   d. _____

   e. _____

2. What are some benefits of providing massage services to hospital staff? One answer is provided.

   a. improved morale _____

   b. _____

   c. _____

   d. _____

   e. _____

   f. _____

3. What are some of the benefits of providing massage to hospital patients?

   a. _____

   b. _____

   c. _____

   d. _____

4. What are the warning signs associated with cancer?

   a. _____

   b. _____

   c. _____

   d. _____

   e. _____

   f. _____

   g. _____

5. Which types of insurance coverage are more likely to pay for massage?

_____

6. Who can determine medical necessity?

_____

7. Which elements should be contained in a prescription for massage?

a. _____

b. _____

c. _____

d. _____

8. Which information is needed from the client to contact the insurance company for verification?

a. _____

_____

b. _____

_____

c. _____

_____

d. _____

_____

e. _____

_____

f. _____

_____

g. _____

_____

h. _____

_____

MULTIPLE CHOICE: Carefully read each statement. Choose the word or phrase that correctly completes the meaning and write the corresponding letter in the blank provided.

1. Healing approaches that regard the entire person, including the spiritual, physical, mental, emotional, social, and environmental rather than just the symptoms, are considered _____.
   a) alternative
   b) integrative
   c) complementary
   d) holistic

2. Combining conventional Western medical practices with alternative and complementary therapies to best benefit a patient's health is _____.
   a) integrative medicine
   b) holistic medicine
   c) mind-body medicine
   d) all of the above

3. Providing massage services to a patient in a hospital requires _____.
   a) special training
   b) a medical license
   c) a physician's referral or prescription
   d) all of the above

4. The most popular and requested modality at many integrative clinics is _____.
   a) Meditation
   b) Physical therapy
   c) Chiropractic
   d) Massage

5. Massage is not performed on an area that is _____.
   a) bleeding
   b) swollen
   c) burned
   d) all of the above

6. A sore that has not healed normally, lumps underneath the arms or in the breasts, and a persistent hoarseness, coughing, or sore throat are _____.
   a) reasons to refer to a doctor
   b) warning signs of cancerv
   c) contraindications for massage
   d) all of the above

7. A massage prescribed by a physician to address a diagnosed condition can be considered a _____.
   a) therapeutic massage
   b) medical massage
   c) wellness massage
   d) all of the above

8. A prescription for massage should contain _____.
   a) diagnosis of the condition
   b) an order for massage therapy services to be performed
   c) the frequency of treatments
   d) all of the above

9. Which type of insurance is more likely to pay for medical massage services?
   a) major medical policies
   b) health maintenance organizations
   c) personal injury claims
   d) Medicare and Medicaid

10. What should a therapist do before providing services to a client with an insurance claim?
    a) perform a thorough assessment
    b) obtain verification from her insurance carrier
    c) contact her doctor for a prescription
    d) refer her to a doctor for a diagnosis

11. Which form must be signed by the client before a therapist can discuss her case with an insurance agent or other medical personnel?
    a) informed consent
    b) medical history form
    c) medical information release form
    d) assignment of benefits form

12. Why is the 1500 Health Insurance Claim form printed in red ink?
    a) to make it easy to read
    b) so it can be read by an optical scanner
    c) to make it easy to find
    d) all of the above

13. What are CPT codes?
    a) a system to categorize medical services
    b) current procedural terminology
    c) a list of allowable fees for medical procedures
    d) all of the above

WORD REVIEW: Write down the meaning of each of the following words. The list can be used as a study guide for this chapter!

agreement for payment form

_____

_____

_____

_____

allopathic medicine

_____

_____

_____

alternative medicine

_____

_____

_____

_____

assignment of benefits form

_____

_____

_____

_____

CAM

_____

_____

_____

_____

complementary medicine

_____

_____

_____

_____

co-pay

_____

_____

_____

_____

CPT codes

_____

_____

_____

_____

1500 Health Insurance Claim form

_____

_____

_____

_____

hospital-based massage

_____

_____

_____

_____

ICD-10 codes

_____

_____

_____

_____

integrative medicine

_____

_____

_____

_____

medical information release form

_____

_____

_____

_____

medical massage

_____

_____

_____

_____

mind-body medicine

_____

_____

_____

_____

NCCAM

_____

_____

_____

_____

NIH

_____

_____

_____

_____

CHAPTER 21

Other Therapeutic Techniques

FILL-IN-THE-BLANK: In the space(s) provided, write the word(s) that correctly complete(s) each statement.

1. A contemporary style of bodywork that uses a specially constructed massage chair was popularized in the 1980s by _____.

2. When practicing hot stone massage, the best type of stones are made of _____.

3. The best stones to use for cold stone therapy are made of _____.

4. When performing hot stone massage on a healthy client, the stones should be heated to _____.

5. The art and science of stimulating certain points on the body (especially the hands and feet) that affect organs or functions in distant parts of the body is known as _____.

6. _____, which preceded reflexology, was developed and popularized by Dr. William Fitzgerald.

7. Reflexology that is practiced on the ears is called _____.

SHORT ANSWER: In the spaces provided, write short answers to the following questions.

1. Which type of lubricant is usually used for chair massage?

   _____

2. Which areas of the body are usually included in a chair massage?

   _____

3. List three reasons learning chair massage is an ideal choice for the massage student or new practitioner.

   a. _____

   b. _____

   c. _____

4. What alerts a reflexologist to places to work on the foot?

   a. _____

   b. _____

5. List two techniques unique to foot reflexology that resemble the movement of an inchworm.

   a. _____

   b. _____

FILL-IN-THE-BLANK: In the space(s) provided, write the word(s) that correctly complete(s) each statement.

1. A traditional Chinese medical practice whereby the skin is punctured with needles at specific points for therapeutic purposes is known as _____.

2. According to Traditional Chinese Medicine, the fundamental substance of existence is _____.

3. In Eastern philosophies, the opposing yet complementary aspects of existence are represented by _____ and _____.

4. In Eastern Asia, the vast web of invisible energy that intertwines all creation is known as _____.

5. **MATCHING:** Arrange the following words in two columns. In the first column, list words that correspond to *yin*. In the second column, write the words that correspond to *yang* adjacent to the contrasting word in the *yin* column. An example is provided.

active	back of the body	cold	contracting
dark	day	deficient	excessive
expanding	forceful	front of the body	high
hot	inner body	inside	light
low	lower body	night	outer body
outside	overactive	passive	underactive
upper body	weak		

YIN	YANG
cold	hot
_____	_____
_____	_____
_____	_____
_____	_____
_____	_____
_____	_____
_____	_____
_____	_____
_____	_____
_____	_____
_____	_____
_____	_____

6. In the following exercise, list the names of the 12 organ meridians, whether each organ is yin or yang, and the element related to it. The first row is provided.

	Organ/meridian	Yin or Yang	Element
a.	lung	yin	metal
b.			
c.			
d.			
e.			
f.			
g.			
h.			
i			
j			
k.			
l.			

FILL-IN-THE-BLANK: In the space(s) provided, write the word(s) that correctly complete(s) each statement.

1. The two basic kinds of Qi are _____ and _____ .

2. In traditional Chinese medicine (TCM), two common methods of assessment are

   a. _____

   b. _____

3. According to ancient philosophy, qi manifests itself as five interrelated elements. They are

   a. _____   d. _____

   b. _____   e. _____

   c. _____

4. Qi moves through the body in specific channels called _____ .

5. There are _____ bilateral channels that relate to the organs.

6. Along these channels are small areas of high conductivity called _____ _____ .

7. Several treatment systems that incorporate various manipulations (not needles) on acupoints are collectively called _____ .

8. The Japanese system of finger pressure massage is called _____ .

9. A technique in TCM of burning an herb, such as mugwort, over an acupoint or on an acupuncture needle is called _____ .

10. A form of Chinese bodywork that is based in TCM and incorporates methods to move energy along the meridians is _____ .

11. In the practice of Zen shiatsu, the primary assessment technique is _____ .

12. A traditional medicine system that originated in India and that uses herbs, massage, and diet as treatment forms is called _____ .

13. A form of energetic bodywork that originated in Japan, in which the practitioner uses mantras and intention to channel energy rather than actual touch is called _____ .

14. _____ was created by Dr. Randolph Stone.

15. A form of energetic bodywork that is popular among nurses and is practiced in hospitals that seeks to balance the human energy field by the practitioner moving their hands near but not on the client's body is called _____ .

MULTIPLE CHOICE: Carefully read each statement. Choose the word or phrase that correctly completes the meaning and write the corresponding letter in the blank provided.

1. David Palmer developed the first specially designed massage chair in _____ _____ .

   a) 1885   c) 1986
   b) 1969   d) 1994

2. Which of the following strokes are not appropriate for chair massage? _____
   a) gliding   c) compression
   b) deep pressure   d) percussion

3. The bodywork practice in which points in the hands or feet are massaged _____ to affect organs or other parts of the body is _____ .
   a) acupuncture   c) reflexology
   b) shiatsu   d) Reiki

4. Acupuncture and TCM originated _____ years ago.
   a) 2,500
   c) 1,000
   b) 5,000
   d) 500

   _____

5. Traditional Chinese medicine was originally conceived by _____.
   a) Taoist monks
   c) the Yellow Emperor
   b) the king's physicians
   d) tribal shamans

   _____

6. According to Eastern philosophy, the fundamental substance of which everything is composed is _____.
   a) atoms
   c) the five elements
   b) yin and yang
   d) qi

   _____

7. Which of the following is yin?
   a) extrovert
   c) contracting
   b) masculine
   d) active

   _____

8. Which of the following is an example of the interaction of yin and yang?
   a) metabolism
   c) breathing
   b) digestion
   d) all of the above

   _____

9. Which of the following is not one of the five elements of traditional Chinese medicine?
   a) earth
   c) fire
   b) water
   d) air

   _____

10. Which element do the spleen, stomach, yellow, and worry correspond to?
    a) fire
    c) water
    b) earth
    d) metal

    _____

11. The _____ meridian starts on the face and ends on the little toe.
    a) bladder
    c) stomach
    b) gallbladder
    d) kidney

    _____

12. In TCM, there are _____ bilateral organ-related meridians.
    a) six
    c) twelve
    b) eight
    d) twenty-four

    _____

13. A primary form of assessment in Chinese medicine is _____. _____
    a) blood pressure
    b) pulse
    c) posture
    d) temperature

14. A form of Chinese bodywork that is grounded in traditional Chinese _____
    medicine is _____.
    a) tuina
    b) shiatsu
    c) anmo
    d) ayurveda

15. A Japanese form of bodywork that uses finger pressure to stimulate or _____
    balance qi flow is _____.
    a) tuina
    b) anmo
    c) shiatsu
    d) Reiki

16. Energy vortexes aligned along front of the spine are called _____. _____
    a) acupoints
    b) chakras
    c) marma points
    d) all of the above

WORD REVIEW: Write down the meaning of each of the following words and phrases. The list can be used as a study guide for this chapter!

acupoint

_____

_____

_____

acupressure

_____

_____

_____

Ayurveda

_____

_____

_____

bioenergy

_____

_____

_____

chair massage

_____

_____

_____

chakra

_____

_____

_____

ki

_____

_____

_____

moxibustion

_____

_____

_____

organ meridian

_____

_____

_____

pulse diagnosis

_____

_____

_____

reflexology

_____

_____

_____

Reiki

_____

_____

_____

shiatsu

_____

_____

_____

therapeutic touch

_____

_____

_____

traditional Chinese medicine (TCM)

_____

_____

_____

tuina

_____

_____

_____

yang

_____

_____

_____

yin

_____

_____

_____

CHAPTER
22 Business Practices

SHORT ANSWER: In the spaces provided, write short answers to the following questions.

1. When does business planning begin?

   _____

2. When does business planning end?

   _____

3. Name four important parts of business planning.

   a. _____

   b. _____

   c. _____

   d. _____

4. List three criteria that differentiate an employee from an independent contractor. Give examples of each.

   a. _____

   _____

   _____

   b. _____

   _____

   _____

c. _____

_____

_____

5. What are the four common types of business operations?

a. _____

b. _____

c. _____

d. _____

FILL-IN-THE-BLANK: In the space(s) provided, write the word(s) that correctly complete(s) each statement.

1. A short general statement of the main focus of the business is called the _____.

2. Specific, attainable, measurable things or accomplishments that you set and make a commitment to achieve are termed _____.

3. If you are an individual owner of a business and carry all expenses, obligations, liabilities, and assets, you are considered a _____.

4. To establish a _____, a charter must be obtained from the state in which the business operates.

5. Management of a corporation is carried out by a _____.

6. When a business is beginning, the expenses incurred before any revenues are collected are considered _____.

7. The primary reason for the failure of small businesses is _____ _____.

SHORT ANSWER: In the spaces provided, write short answers to the following questions.

1. If your business is a sole proprietorship, who is responsible for any losses or debts?

_____

_____

2. Which zoning requirements must be considered when working out of your own home?

_____

_____

3. List at least three important considerations when buying an established business.

a. _____

b. _____

c. _____

FILL-IN-THE-BLANK: In the space(s) provided, write the word(s) that correctly complete(s) each statement.

1. If a business is operating under a name other than the owner's, a _____ _____ is required.

2. If the business sells products or if services are taxed, a _____ must be obtained from _____.

3. To ensure that the business meets zoning requirements, the _____ _____ should be contacted.

4. An employer identification number must be obtained from the _____ if the business hires employees.

5. The identification number issued to licensed healthcare providers and used when submitting claims to medical insurance companies is called a _____.

6. As a massage business owner, one should have adequate insurance against _____, _____, and _____.

KEY CHOICES: Choose the types of insurance that best fit the description. Write the appropriate key letter next to the stated description in the space provided. The insurance types may be used more than once.

A. automobile insurance   E. liability insurance

B. disability insurance   F. professional liability insurance

C. fire and theft insurance   G. workers' compensation insurance

D. health insurance

_____ 1. protects the person from loss of income because they are unable to work because of long-term illness or injury

_____ 2. helps to cover the cost of medical bills, especially hospitalization, serious injury, or illness

_____ 3. provides medical and liability insurance to the driver and any passengers

_____ 4. is required if you have employees

_____ 5. covers the cost of fixtures, furniture, equipment, products, and supplies

_____ 6. covers costs of injuries and litigation resulting from injuries sustained on the owner's property

_____ 7. covers the medical costs for the employee if they are injured on the job

_____ 8. covers the vehicle and its contents, regardless of who is at fault

_____ 9. protects the therapist from lawsuits filed by a client because of injury or loss that results from negligence or substandard performance

FILL-IN-THE-BLANK: In the space(s) provided, write the word(s) that correctly complete(s) each statement.

1. When setting fees for massage, consider your experience and expertise, _____, and the _____.

2. A summary of all sales and cash receipts/invoices is called an _____.

3. A ledger that records, separates, and classifies business expenditures is called a _____.

SHORT ANSWER: In the spaces provided, write short answers to the following questions.

1. If a massage business is operated out of a home, are all telephone expenses tax deductible?

_____

_____

2. For a self-employed massage practitioner, which three major records should be maintained?

a. _____

b. _____

c. _____

3. Two important reasons for keeping accurate financial records are

a. _____

b. _____

4. Why is it advisable to consult an accountant when preparing taxes?

_____

_____

5. Which name is on the business checking account?

_____

6. Which moneys are deposited in the business account?

_____

7. For which purposes are checks written from the business account?

_____

8. What is the purpose of a petty cash fund?

_____

9. Where does petty cash fund money come from?

_____

10. How long should canceled checks and bank statements be kept for tax purposes?

_____

11. What is included in the income records?

_____

12. Name 10 things that should be included on an income receipt or invoice.

a. _____   g. _____

b. _____   h. _____

c. _____   i. _____

d. _____   j. _____

e. _____   k. _____

f. _____   l. _____

13. How many copies of the invoice should there be, and where do they go?

_____

14. Information that is included in each entry of the disbursement ledger includes

a. _____

b. _____

c. _____

d. _____

e. _____

15. Which receipts should be kept and filed?

_____

16. How long should receipts be kept?

_____

17. When is it necessary to keep an accounts receivable file?

_____

18. A record of money owed to other persons or businesses is kept in an _____ file.

19. Items and equipment that are purchased to be used in the business for an extended time (more than a year) are called _____ .

20. Are the products that are for sale in the business considered business assets?

_____

21. Which information should be kept in a record of business assets?

_____

_____

22. What are two methods of determining business-related automobile expenses?

_____

_____

23. What is usually kept in a client record?

a. _____

b. _____

c. _____

24. What is the importance of an appointment book or scheduling program?

_____

_____

FILL-IN-THE-BLANK: In the space(s) provided, write the word(s) that correctly complete(s) each statement.

1. The business activity done to promote and increase business is called _____ .

2. A segment of the population with similar characteristics that the practitioner might prefer to attract is called the _____ .

3. Most promotional activities are _____ in nature.

4. Any marketing activity that the practitioner must pay for directly is considered _____ .

5. In today's electronic environment, and effective marketing tool is a _____ .

6. The practice of encouraging clients to come back for services repeatedly is known as _____ .

SHORT ANSWER: In the spaces provided, write short answers to the following questions.

1. List five marketing activities.

   a. _____

   b. _____

   c. _____

   d. _____

   e. _____

2. What is the advantage of selecting a target market?

   _____

   _____

3. What are two ways of determining a target market?

   a. _____

   _____

   b. _____

   _____

4. Give four examples of printed promotional materials.

a. _____

b. _____

c. _____

d. _____

5. What should be included on every piece of promotional material?

_____

6. Three Internet platforms that provide businesses and individuals to network with others are

a. _____

b. _____

c. _____

7. What are two objectives of promotional activities?

a. _____

b. _____

8. List four ways to promote business through public relations.

_____

_____

_____

_____

_____

_____

_____

_____

_____

_____

9. What are two main sources for obtaining referrals?

a. _____

b. _____

10. When a satisfied client refers a new person, what should be done?

_____

11. When a healthcare professional refers a client, what should be done?

a. _____

b. _____

c. _____

12. What are the three Rs of referrals?

a. _____

b. _____

c. _____

SHORT ANSWER: In the spaces provided, write short answers to the following questions.

1. Which federal regulations must be observed when operating a massage business with employees?

a. _____

b. _____

c. _____

2. Which state regulations must be observed when operating a massage business?

a. _____

b. _____

c. _____

d. _____

e. _____

MULTIPLE CHOICE: Carefully read each statement. Choose the word or phrase that correctly completes the meaning and write the corresponding letter in the blank provided.

1. A positive self-image means that you _____.
   a) like yourself and what you do
   b) look beautiful
   c) wear expensive clothes
   d) are vain

2. Your public image includes all of the following EXCEPT _____.
   a) appearance
   b) business conduct
   c) expense reports
   d) customer relations

3. Clarifying your business' purpose, stating a mission, setting goals, and determining priorities is called _____.
   a) accounting
   b) business planning
   c) tax preparation
   d) job training

4. A short, general statement of the business's main focus is called a/an _____,
   a) goal
   b) business plan
   c) advertisement
   d) mission statement

5. A business that has one owner is called a _____.
   a) sole proprietorship
   b) partnership
   c) corporation
   d) limited liability company

6. A business that has stockholders is called a
   a) sole proprietorship
   b) partnership
   c) corporation
   d) subsidiary

7. Inadequate capital to cover business expenses and poor choice of location are the main reasons for small business _____.
   a) expansion
   b) insurance
   c) failure
   d) advertising

8. When buying an existing business, make sure it is _____.
   a) well established
   b) reputable
   c) in a good location
   d) all of the above

9. The insurance that covers costs of injuries occurring on your property and any resulting litigation is called _____ insurance.
   a) disability
   b) liability
   c) homeowners'
   d) workers' compensation

10. Insurance that protects the therapist from lawsuits filed by a client because of injury or loss from negligence or poor execution of a professional skill is called _____ insurance.
    a) property
    b) disability
    c) compensation
    d) malpractice

11. Insurance that covers the medical costs for employees injured on the job is called _____ insurance.
    a) workers' compensation
    b) malpractice
    c) liability
    d) disability

12. A ledger that separates and classifies every business expenditure is called a/an _____.
    a) inventory
    b) disbursement record
    c) profit/loss statement
    d) balance sheet

13. All of the following are business expenses EXCEPT _____.
    a) rent
    b) supplies
    c) advertising
    d) owner's salary

14. The marketing activity done in return for direct payment is called _____.
    a) publicity
    b) advertising
    c) bartering
    d) referral

15. Developing personal and professional contacts for the purpose of giving and receiving support and sharing information is called _____.
    a) hobnobbing
    b) networking
    c) advertising
    d) promotions

16. The best and least expensive way to create new business is through _____.
    a) referrals
    b) advertising
    c) public speaking
    d) client retention

17. Social Security and unemployment compensation are two regulations of the _____ government.
    a) state
    b) federal
    c) county
    d) city

18. Sales taxes, licenses, and workers' compensation are required by
    _____ government.   _____
    a) state   c) county
    b) federal   d) city

19. A person hired on as her own boss is called a/an _____.   _____
    a) employee   c) independent contractor
    b) bookkeeper   d) receptionist

WORD REVIEW: Write down the meaning of each of the following words. The list can be used as a study guide for this chapter!

accounts payable

_____

_____

_____

_____

accounts receivable

_____

_____

_____

_____

advertising

_____

_____

_____

_____

bank account reconciliation

_____

_____

_____

_____

bank statement

_____

_____

_____

_____

bookkeeping

_____

_____

_____

_____

business assets

_____

_____

_____

_____

business checking account

_____

_____

_____

_____

business expenditures

_____

_____

_____

_____

business goals

_____

_____

_____

_____

business license

_____

_____

_____

_____

client file

_____

_____

_____

_____

client retention

_____

_____

_____

_____

corporation

_____

_____

_____

_____

cost of goods

_____

_____

_____

_____

DBA

_____

_____

_____

_____

direct mail

_____

_____

_____

_____

disbursement ledger

_____

_____

_____

_____

EIN

_____

_____

_____

_____

fictitious name statement

_____

_____

_____

_____

goals

_____

_____

_____

_____

income ledger

_____

_____

_____

_____

independent contractor

_____

_____

_____

_____

inventory

_____

_____

_____

_____

invoice

_____

_____

_____

_____

LLC

_____

_____

_____

_____

limited liability company

_____

_____

_____

_____

marketing

_____

_____

_____

_____

massage license

_____

_____

_____

_____

mileage log

_____

_____

_____

_____

mission statement

_____

_____

_____

_____

outcalls

_____

_____

_____

_____

partnership

_____

_____

_____

_____

personal draw

_____

_____

_____

_____

petty cash fund

_____

_____

_____

_____

professional liability insurance

_____

_____

_____

_____

provider's number

_____

_____

_____

_____

record keeping

_____

_____

_____

_____

referral

_____

_____

_____

_____

Schedule C

_____

_____

_____

_____

Schedule SE

_____

_____

_____

_____

self-employed

_____

_____

_____

_____

sole proprietor

_____

_____

_____

_____

start-up costs

_____

_____

_____

_____

target market

_____

_____

_____

_____

tax deductible

_____

_____

_____

_____

word-of-mouth advertising

_____

_____

_____

_____

zoning regulations

_____

_____

_____

_____

NOTES

NOTES

NOTES

NOTES

NOTES